Medical Fasting and Therapeutics

Dr. MORTAGY RASHED

ISBN: 1501011820

ISBN 13: 9781501011825

Library of Congress Control Number: XXXXXX (If applicable)

LCCN Imprint Name: City and State (If applicable)

Introduction

The purpose of therapeutic fasting is the promotion and restoration of health. It is associated with experimental and physiological fasting in the sense that studies of the latter provide the knowledge and information that make therapeutic fasting possible.

Therapeutic fasting is not the result of any particular new scientific discovery; rather, it has proceeded to its present development as the result of centuries of experimentation, observation, and study. It is today the culmination of a large number of scientific investigations and discoveries that have reached their climax during the past century. Fasting for therapeutic purposes is thus an important, though in popular conception, almost unknown, phase of the modern science of medicine, and as such, it is the subject of our present inquiry and analysis.

Let's also keep in mind that fasting is only one part of the total health-supporting program that we call natural hygiene.

Health results from healthful living. No matter how successful a fasting experience may be, it needs to be followed by a consistently healthy lifestyle. The requirements of health must continue to be provided, especially in the areas of diet, environment, activity, and psychology.

People who undertake a fast in a supervised setting tend to achieve health more quickly than those who attempt changes without a fast. The intensive health education plus the emotional support they receive during their stay results in increased compliance with dietary and lifestyle recommendations.

When individuals try to make significant dietary changes without the benefit of a fasting experience, they often become frustrated. The transition to a healthful eating pattern can make them feel sick. Symptoms such as fatigue, nausea, vomiting, diarrhea, abdominal pain and bloating, joint pain, headaches, skin rashes, irritability, depression, etc. are just a few of the common problems that can arise as the body attempts to eliminate toxins, metabolic byproducts, etc. and adjust physiologically to a health-promoting diet.

It is difficult to get people to practice new healthful-living habits for long unless they begin to experience some benefits immediately. Changes that may take months (or even years) with careful eating may occur much more quickly if a properly supervised fast is utilized. This is an important consideration because once people begin to realize their health potential, they become likely candidates for a lifelong commitment to healthful living.

CHAPTER 1

Fasting in history

When the principles of religions appeared in the world little by little, their leaders and priests took the fasting condition for worship as a means to get closer to the gods. In ancient Egypt and Mesopotamia and the rest of the centers of ancient civilization, people were required to enroll in the service of the temple and to fast seven full days. They were not to eat then —only a few doses of water—and the duration of the fasting sometimes extended to forty-two days.

The Persians trained their children to fast since early childhood in order to grow up strong and endure difficult tasks. The Greeks also imposed fasting in their beliefs.

Fasting-known religions, Sabine's and Manichaeism and Abrahamic and Buddhists, that in the law Aharanyen, known as saúbh, which is a religion based on reverence, the planets imposed on them to fast for thirty days in honor of the moon and the fast was not to stop for food and beverages from sunrise to sunset, they were fast for nine days in honor of the buyer and seven days in honor of the lord of the sun; the majorities do not eat meat or what comes out of the animals, and they do not drink alcohol..

In the law of fasting. Albarhamaan imposed fasting on the layer of the priests during the early seasons of the year: on the first day and the fourteenth day of every lunar month. Buddhists imposed fasting from sunrise to sunset four days of every lunar month, which necessitated comfort and deprived them from engaging in any business. There is a kind of Buddhist that practices long-term fasting within the year. This separates the soul from the material body and makes it indomitable. In China, India, and Japan, the likes of the great long-term fasting worshipers who endured these calls of the sons of Buddhism and Abrahamic beliefs are surprising. It is worth mentioning here that Gandhi practiced extended fasting as a means of protest against English policy in an effort to liberate his country, India.

Fasting in Judaism:

 According to the first paragraph of chapter nine of Nehemiah, one of the historical books of the Old Testament, there is evidence that Jews fasted on the twenty-fourth day of the seventh month of the Hebrew calendar. And understand what is stated in the book of Zechariah: after they left for Babylon, they fasted for days. Many other periodic painful memories in their history were all so-called "fast" ones. There was no Hebrew month in which they occurred without incident.

Fasting in Christianity:

Nothing in the known text of the Gospels implies obligatory fasting, but it is mentioned and praised and considered a cult. It was never for showing off. Then the heads of the church initiated a broad spectrum of fasting, creating a disagreement between the sects and denominations, including fasting from meat, fish, eggs, and milk. Now Lent has some Christian denominations abstaining from food and drink from midnight to noon, or twelve hours, for forty consecutive days. Other communities fast for fifty days, omitting eating animal products, which they would otherwise be permitted to eat.

It seems that fasting was known to the Arabs before Islam.

Fasting in Islam:

In Islam, the practice is to abstain from food, drink, and other foods, not breaking the fast from dawn to sunset. The fasting month of Ramadan, the corner of the five pillars of Islam, imposed by God for a Muslim resident of the rational and non-patient, he says: ((O ye who believe! Fasting is prescribed to you as it was prescribed to those before you, that ye may (learn)self-restraint, fasting for a fixed number of days; but if any of you is ill, or on the journey ,the prescribed number (should be made up)from days later. For those who can do it (with hardship), is a ransom, the feeding of one that is indigent. But he that will give more, of his own free will,-it is

better for him, and it is better for you that ye fast, if ye only knew))
(Albaqarah 183-184).

There are many sayings of the prophet about fasting,

Abu Hurairah (May Allah is pleased with him) reported:

The Messenger of Allah said, "When any one of you is observing Saum (fasting) on a day, he should neither indulge in obscene language nor should he raise the voice; and if anyone reviles him or tries to quarrel with him he should say: 'I am observing fast.'"

[Al-Bukhari and Muslim].

Narrated Abu Huraira:

The Prophet said, "Allah said: The Fast is for Me and I will give the reward for it, as he (the one who observes the fast) leaves his sexual desire, food and drink for My Sake. Fasting is a screen (from Hell) and there are two pleasures for a fasting person, one at the time of breaking his fast, and the other at the time when he will meet his Lord. And the smell of the mouth of a fasting person is better in Allah's Sight than the smell of musk." (See Hadith No. 128, Vol. 3).

Muslims remained (and remain until this time) committed to perform the hajj in the fasting month of Ramadan and to do so in the form imposed by God and the prophet, enacted without change or switch, believing that corner of the great religion of Islam.

The types of volunteer fasting in Islam are:

1 - Fasting for the six days of Shawwal

2 - Fasting the day of Arafat (nine of Dhul-Hiijah)

3 - Fasting and Tasso's Ashura (the ninth and tenth of Muharram)

4 - A lot of fasting in Sha'ban.

5 - Fasting during the sacred months (November, December, Muharram, and Rajab)

6 - Fasting three days every month

7 - Fasting on Mondays and Thursdays

8 - Fasting on the fast day from breakfast on

CHAPTER 2

Chemical and organic changes during fasting

Abstinence from food may mean missing one meal, or it may mean going without food until death results from starvation. Missing one meal produces no organic or chemical changes in the body; in starvation, many changes occur. It is necessary to know that various changes occur at different stages of the period of abstinence, and that the changes at different stages are of different, even opposite, character. For example, in women and female animals, atrophy of the mammary glands is seen in starvation, but in fasting, there is only a loss of fat. In the early stages of abstinence in young guinea pigs, the pancreas, like the other internal organs, is in general more resistant to loss of weight. Pancreatic losses in the early stages of abstinence are relatively slight, while in advanced stages, that is, in starvation, pancreatic loss (atrophy) is extreme, being, as a rule, relatively greater than that of the entire body. Many examples of similar differences will be given throughout the pages of this book.

There is naturally and necessarily a loss of weight when humans or animals cease to eat, and if food is abstained from long enough, death results from too great of a loss. In discussing the differences *between fasting and starving,* we made use of Margulies's three stages of the inanition period—from the omission of the first meal until its ending in death. In general, in both birds and mammals, the loss of weight is greatest during the first third of the inanition period, least in the second third, and intermediate in the last third, although this final acceleration of loss is variable or even absent.

In all animals, from worms to man, the various organs and tissues of the body differ significantly in their rates of loss while fasting and starving. In general, it may be said that most of the soft tissues of the body lose weight during a fast, but they lose at varying rates. Instead of a uniform wasting of the body's resources, biologically vital organs are sustained at the expense of less important ones.

Structural changes during fasting are largely those that result from loss of weight. At death from starvation, the amount of weight lost may amount to 50–60 percent. No such losses are registered in a fast. As I pointed out before, individual organs or tissues show a very unequal emaciation: some are living at the expense of others.

It is interesting to note some of the losses and changes that occur during a fast. In death by starvation, the following losses have been observed by some investigators:

Fat	91%
Spleen	63%
Muscle	30%
Blood	17%
Liver	56%
Nerves	???

Yeo's physiology gives the estimated losses that occur in death from starvation as:

Fat	97%
Spleen	63%
Muscle	30%
Blood	17%
Liver	56%
Nerves	000

According to Chossat, the losses sustained by the various tissues in starvation are as follows:

Fat   93%

Nerves   2%

Muscles   43%

Pancreas 64%

Liver   52%

Spleen   70%

Blood   75%

Chossat's table was made from animal experimentation and agrees very well with the observations of others, except in the loss of blood. Others have given this as less than 20 percent. The *International Encyclopedia,* under "fasting," gives a table showing the losses sustained by an animal while fasting for thirteen days. This table gives the loss of blood for this time as 17 percent and the loss to the brain and nerves as none.

It will be observed that during the fast the tissues do not all waste at an equal rate: those that are not necessary are utilized most rapidly; those least basic, less rapidly; and those most important, not at all at first and only slowly at the last. Nature always favors the most vital organs. The fat disappears first, and then the other tissues disappear in the inverse order of their usefulness. The essential tissues obtain their nourishment from the less important by enzyme action, a process which has been termed *autolysis*.

These tables show that the brain and nervous system continue intact (retain their structural and functional integrity) until the last and retain the inherent power to maintain their nutrition unimpaired—although every other tissue has wasted beyond repair—and that the blood, even in the most extreme cases, does not show extraordinary depletion.

Such physiological facts would seem to argue that nerve and blood supply throughout the body are virtually standard during a fast, and that the human body is, in reality, a veritable organization of assailable food elements dominated by a self-maintaining intelligence that is capable of preserving relative structural integrity and physiologic functional balance, even when all food is withheld for considerable intervals.

Only in a very special sense does the body "start eating itself" when one begins to fast. It never consumes its tissues indiscriminately, but, true to its rule of always favoring its most vital organs, it uses up the least useful tissues first. Selective action is exercised from the beginning, and the most rigid economy is exercised in appropriating its food reserves in sustaining the heart, lungs, brain, nerves, and other vital organs. Even the respiratory muscles are more carefully guarded than the other muscles of the skeleton.

Diagram 1 shows the percentage of the total loss of the body borne by each organ in death by starvation, while diagram 2 shows the percentage of loss in each organ under the same circumstances. These tables also include the proportion that the loss in each bears to the weight of a similar animal killed in good condition.

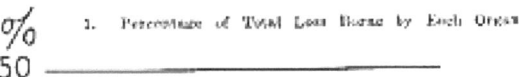

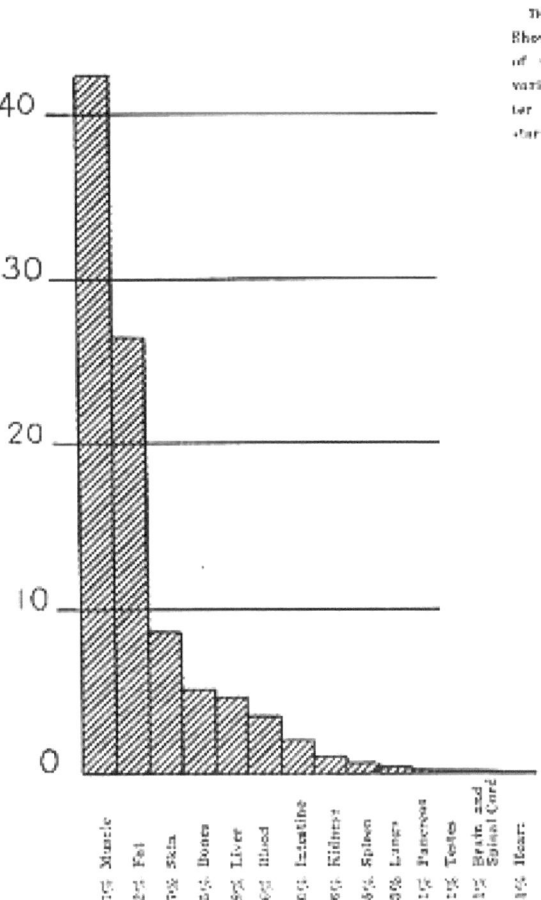

DIAGRAM 1.
Showing the loss
of weight of the
various organs af-
ter death from
starvation.

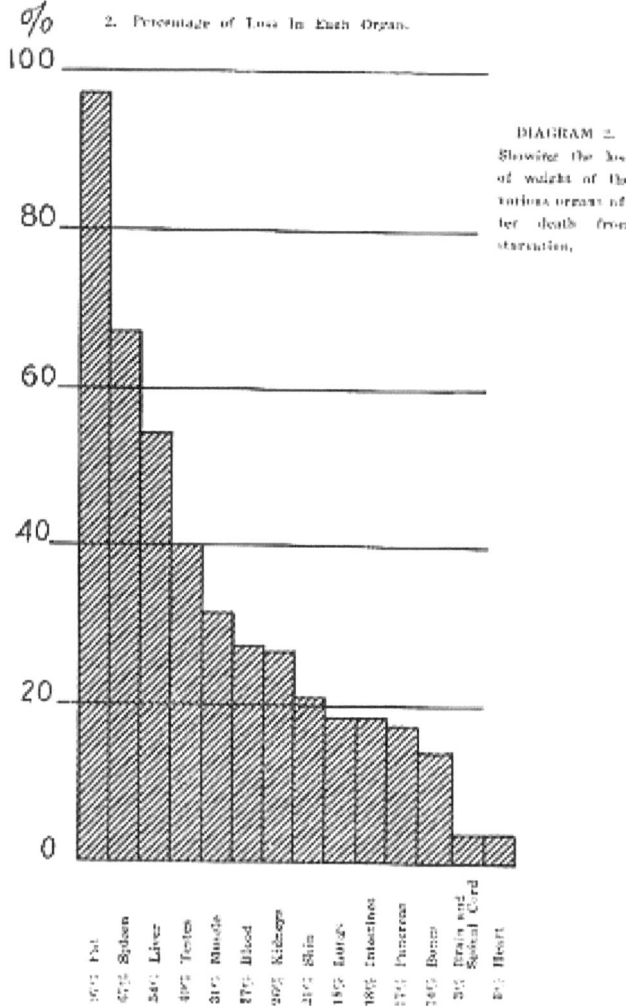

2. Percentage of Loss In Each Organ.

DIAGRAM 2.
Showing the loss
of weight of the
various organs af-
ter death from
starvation.

The careful student will bear in mind that most of the actual tissue loss shown by these tables occurred in the last third of the inanition period—the period of starvation proper—and did not occur during the fasting period.

While table 1 shows that the musculature of the body supplies the greatest loss of weight, the actual loss to the muscles only reaches 21 percent of the total muscular substance (chiefly the superficial muscles), while, though the actual proportion of the weight lost is less, 97 percent of the fat present is used up. The other organs that lose much of their weight are the spleen (with 67 percent), the liver (with 54 percent), and the testes (with 40 percent). The central nervous tissue and the heart supply only 0.1 percent of the total loss and 3 percent of their actual substance.

A closer and more detailed view of the losses to the more vital organs and tissues will help us to better understand the subjects we are dealing with here.

The difference between Islamic fasting and starvation (medical fasting)

The definition of Islamic religious fasting is: to refrain from eating, drinking, and having sexual intercourse from dawn to sunset with intention.

The medical definition of fasting (starvation) is the partial or total abstinence from eating food and drinks together or eating food only for a period of time.

Benefits of starvation (medical fasting):

This can be summarized in the following points:

1 - To provide comfort to all organs of the body.

2 - To remove toxins and waste from the body.

3 - To renew tissue cells.

Indeed, experiments conducted on humans were performed on dogs in the laboratory at the University of Chicago, and the findings were published in the *Journal of Metabolic Research,* showing that habitually for 30-40 days gives an increase in the amount of metabolism from 5-6%, and if we know that the shortage in the degree of metabolic rate is a manifestation of aging, then we know that fasting increases the rate of metabolism in the body and eliminates the accumulated toxins and absorbs the dead tissues of the weak tissue and replaces it with a new .

Fasting is good for its own sake and to achieve the benefits of the believer and the spiritual pleasure and happiness in this world and the hereafter.

These benefits and the benefits realized each taxpayer healthy residents, and who fast without discomfort excess of the people of licenses who can eat my meal breakfast and suhoor like healthy, and there is no scientific research -

far - was conducted on fasting healthy, in ordinary circumstances, however one of two things: either a lack of the effect of fasting on the physiology and body composition in any amount is dangerous to the body or cause harm to achieving most of the diseases., it shows a definite interest in some of these jobs, improve some components of the body and physiology in aging, during pregnancy, breast-feeding while traveling, and even research proved that fasting helps in curing some diseases.

And thus the fast remains useful for most patients, travelers, and pieties of fasting, and be achieving them of the benefits and benefits a bit too much, which does not teach. Fasting for patients, travelers and pieties is the first and most useful, unless weaken self-bear hardship, hit it or infects the body.

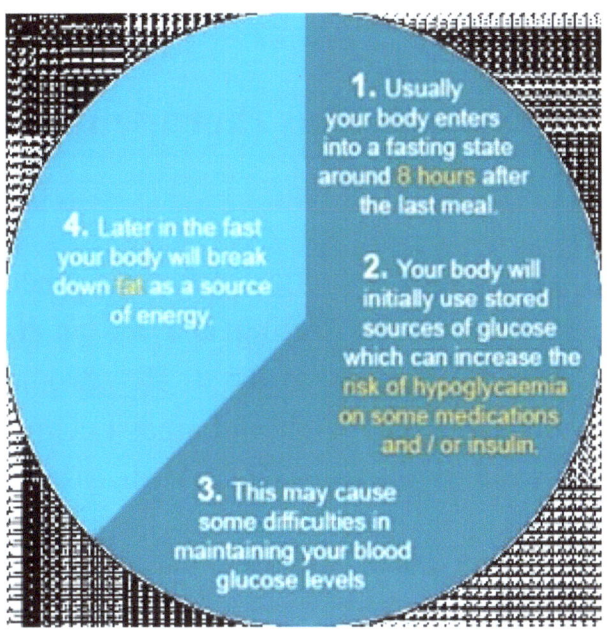

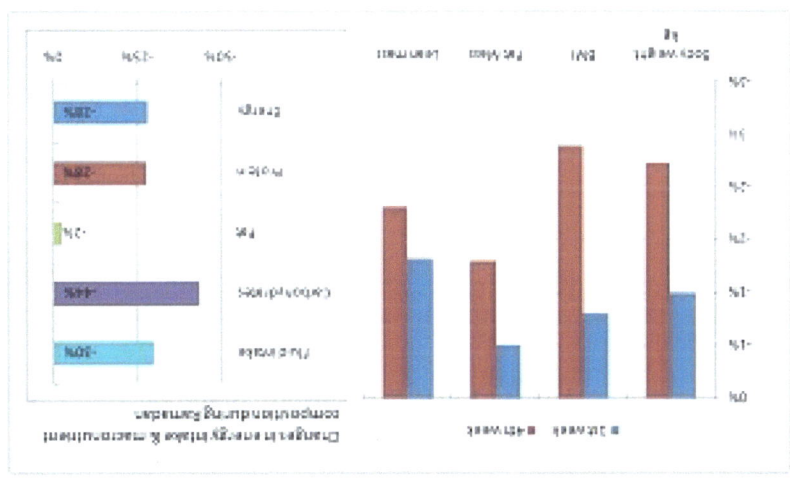

Changes in body composition (left) as a consequence of four weeks of Ramadan fasting at the given (self-selected) macronutrient amounts (right) in rugby players (data calculated based on Bouhlel 2008).

CHAPTER 3

Fasting means therapeutic

After the spread of Islam and the practice of fasting, when the Islamic many nations explain the virtues of the fasting and its benefits, "described the Muslim doctor (Ibn Sina) fasting to treat all chronic diseases, and a description Muslim doctors in the tenth and atheist century (AD) to fast for three weeks to heal from smallpox, and HIV disease, during Napoleon's occupation of Egypt was the application of fasting in hospitals for the treatment of venereal diseases."

The Renaissance in Europe, calling for scientists to take people by reducing overeating and left to indulge in pleasures, drink and fasting propose to mitigate the unbridled desires. In Germany, he found a doctor (Frederick Hoffman) (1660-1842 AD) that fasting (meant starvation sustained is known as fasting Medical) shall be appointed to deal with epilepsy, ulcers and cancers of blood and cataract (a), which affects the eyes and tumors of the gums and bleeding and ulcers palpebral, as announced Patients are advised that in any disease, not to eat something.

Russia, doctors to reach a similar result, in the eighteenth and nineteenth centuries. It has offered Dr. (Petervenya Minoves) from Moscow State University report published in the year 1769 it advised patients to stop for food during the total period of the disease. He reasoned that by saying: "Fasting gives the stomach a rest period enables the patient to digest properly when it recovers, and goes back to eating again," then Dr. (b. C. Spassky), a professor at the University of Moscow, for success in treatment (relapsing fever) fasting, said: "The fast growing processors allowed to happen in the inside of the body, without interference from the outside, and this is in fact the treatment of chronic diseases."

The nineteenth century, declared Russian doctor (Zeeland) that fasting may impact positively on the nervous system of the patient, as affected quite a bit to digest and blood in general, he wrote: Fasting allows the body to relax and then resume his routine with renewed vigor.

The United States, fasting grew attention as a treatment for patients; this has been within the last century. Was treated by Dr. (Edward Dewey) a century ago fasting both disorders and infectious intestinal disease and ascites, and numerous infections, in addition to physical weakness and sagging. He thought that the rest of the food—not food—that restored the nervous system, while the food for the patient caused severely strained as much stress caused by work tired, and emphasizes that the food during the illness, the patient becomes vain.

There has been a proliferation of medical clinics in many countries of the world—east and west—that treat diseases through the use of fasting.

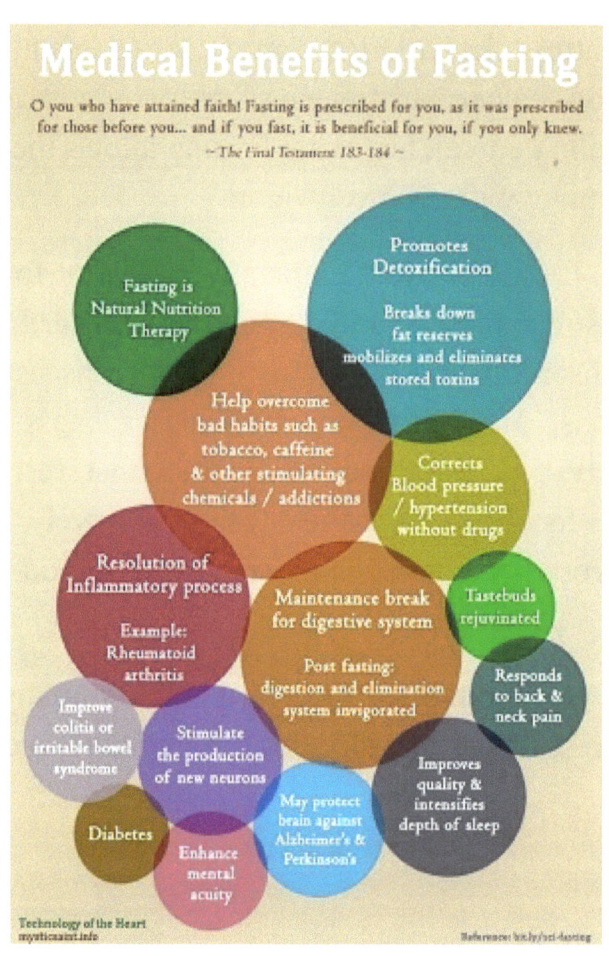

Medical Benefits of Fasting

O you who have attained faith! Fasting is prescribed for you, as it was prescribed
for those before you... and if you fast, it is beneficial for you, if you only knew.
~ The Final Testament 183-184 ~

Fasting is
Natural Nutrition
Therapy

Promotes
Detoxification

Breaks down
fat reserves
mobilizes and eliminates
stored toxins

Help overcome
bad habits such as
tobacco, caffeine
& other stimulating
chemicals / addictions

Corrects
Blood pressure
/ hypertension
without drugs

Resolution of
Inflammatory process

Example:
Rheumatoid
arthritis

Maintenance break
for digestive system

Post fasting:
digestion and elimination
system invigorated

Tastebuds
rejuvinated

Responds
to back &
neck pain

Improve
colitis or
irritable bowel
syndrome

Stimulate
the production
of new neurons

May protect
brain against
Alzheimer's &
Perkinson's

Improves
quality &
intensifies
depth of sleep

Diabetes

Enhance
mental
acuity

Technology of the Heart
mysticsaint.info

Reference: bit.ly/sci-fasting

CHAPTER 4

Fasting and modern scientific research

The development and evolution of the forms of human pathology are governed by the physiological and chemical reactions that are taking place.

Anything that induces such reactions plays a role in determining the state of human health.

Whenever food is withheld from consumption beyond the usual period in the case of man or other animals, there are certain changes in the functions, chemical reactions, and life processes of the cells and tissues. It is these changes that give fasting its therapeutic properties. By considering the physiological reactions to fasting, we can gain an understanding of the reasons that determine its therapeutic value.

Of great importance among the physiological effects of fasting is juvenescence—the acquiring of fresh vitality and the renewal of youthful characteristics to the cells and tissues of the body.

Evidence of such regeneration comes from many areas and is particularly important with respect to experimental work done with the various forms of lower animal life. Such work should then be given our first consideration.

The British scientist by the name of Prof. Huxley has carried out experiments with young planarians, more commonly known as earthworms.

He fed an entire colony of these worms their usual foods. One of the worms was isolated from the rest and fasted at periodic intervals. In all other respects, its diet and mode of life were similar to those of the other worms. The isolated worm lived, while nineteen generations of worms in the colony passed away.

Prof. Child, of the University of Chicago, likewise has used worms to determine the effects of fasting. He took a group of small flatworms, which had grown old and infirmed, and fasted them for months, until they had been reduced to a minimum size.

Then he started feeding them again, and as they grew back to their normal size, they were just as young, from a physiological standpoint, as they ever were.

In his *Senescence and Rejuvenescence*, Prof. Child remarks: "Partial starvation inhibits senescence. The starveling is brought back from an advanced age to the beginning of postembryonic life; it is almost reborn."

Other experiments, conducted by F. Schultz, have shown that those hydras are rejuvenated by fasting, the animals reverting back to an embryonic state.

At the University of Chicago, one insect, the typical life span of which is one day, was fasted the nucleus. Morphologically, therefore, the cells composing the entire organism assumed a more youthful condition.

They resembled more the embryonic cells in this respect, and this may account for the expansive growth which they displayed under the proper nutritive regime."

One of the characteristics of old age is a decrease in the metabolic rate. It is interesting to note, in this connection, that fasting produces rejuvenation by inducing a permanent increase in the metabolic rate.

In experiments conducted at the Hull Biological Laboratory of the University of Chicago, both dogs and humans were fasted for extended periods.

In fasts of from thirty to forty days, a 5–6 percent increase in the metabolic rate was observed.

Of course, rejuvenation does not occur in man to the extent that it does in the lowest forms of animal life. However, the effects of rejuvenescence are nevertheless very noticeable in the case of human fasting.

Dr. Carlson and Dr. Kunde, of the department of physiology in the University of Chicago, placed a forty-year-old man on a fourteen-day fast. At the end of the fast, his tissues were in the same physiological condition as those of a seventeen-year-old youth. In reference to fasting Dr. Kunde remarks: "It is evident that where the initial weight was reduced by 45 percent, and subsequently restored by healthy diet, approximately one-half of the restored body is made up of new protoplasm. In this there is rejuvenescence." It may also be pointed out that quite possibly much of the remaining part of the body not lost in this process undergoes significant changes of rejuvenescence as a result of fasting.

The outward manifestations of regeneration are quite noticeable in many cases of fasting. The rejuvenating effect upon the skin, in particular, is significant. Lines and wrinkles become less apparent, and blotches, discolorations, and pimples tend to disappear.

In the words of Dr. Shelton: "The skin becomes more youthful, acquires a better color and better texture. The eyes clear up and become brighter. One looks younger. The visible rejuvenation in the skin is matched by manifest evidences of similar but invisible rejuvenescence throughout the body.

On the fast, the assimilative powers of the body are increased. This is shown both in the improvement of the blood during the fast and the rapid assimilation of food after the fast.

Patients who suffer from conditions such as anemia, with either an insufficiency of red blood cells or an excess of white cells, are generally normalized by fasting.

In some cases, fasting has brought about an increase in the number of erythrocytes from only one million to the regular five million counts. The explanation lies in the improvement in assimilation that the fast affords.

The iron and other elements that are stored in the body are taken up by the blood and used. Prior to fasting, general physiological inefficiency prevented this.

Perhaps this also explains why dental decay is often arrested during the fast. In some cases, teeth that were loose become firmly fixed in their sockets while fasting, and swollen, inflamed and bleeding gums were also restored to health.

The improvement in assimilation during the fast actually brings about recovery of particular "deficiency" diseases.

Assimilation after the fast is at the highest possible level. Kagan observed that after rabbits were fasted seventeen days, they gained 56 percent in weight on a diet which, under usual conditions, would barely be sufficient to maintain a state of equilibrium. People, who are chronically underweight in spite of eating very heavily, return to the normal level after a fast, even though large quantities of food are not taken.

The improved assimilation enables the body to utilize more of its food intake.

It may be mentioned that it is really a normalization of assimilation that occurs on a fast.

Patients who fast to rid themselves of excessive weight may gain weight to normal after the fast, but that is usually where the increase ends if nutrition is proper.

Thus, both people who assimilate too much of food intake and those who assimilate too little are helped by fasting.

During a fast, the necessary work done by the organs is reduced to the lowest possible minimum. As there is no further intake of food, assimilation in the body only involves the redistribution of the elements already stored there. Thus, the organs are given a chance to recuperate and restore their vital powers.

Associated with physiological rest of an organ is increased elimination. This, according to some observers, is the most important advantage of fasting. Part of the energy that should normally be devoted to the work of assimilation may, during a fast, be used to expel the accumulations of waste and toxins.

Decomposing food in the digestive tract, which is often a significant source of toxins, is quickly eliminated.

The entire alimentary canal becomes almost free from bacteria. The nourishment of cells on a fast is first derived from the less essential tissues and portions of impaired and diseased tissue. The surplus material on hand is utilized first. The effusions, dropsically swellings, fat, infiltrations, etc., are absorbed with great rapidity on a fast.

The body thus gradually releases itself from a former burden of superfluous and waste material. Increased elimination of toxins is noted on the very first days of the fast. The breath becomes very offensive, and the skin may also emit an offensive odor, possibly because of greater eliminative effort on the part of both the lungs and skin.

Catarrhal eliminations usually increase during the early days of the fast, until toward the end of the fast, elimination is completed, and recovery occurs.

The toxicity of the urine is increased, perhaps due to greater elimination via the kidneys. In some cases, considerable waste material is lost through the process of vomiting.

Of course, each of these symptoms does not occur in all cases, but there is always some outward indication of increased elimination.

The primary elimination, however, brought about simply by internal absorption and autolysis, is not apparent in outward reactions, except perhaps the loss of weight and general weakness.

CHAPTER 5

The effect of fasting on gastroenterology

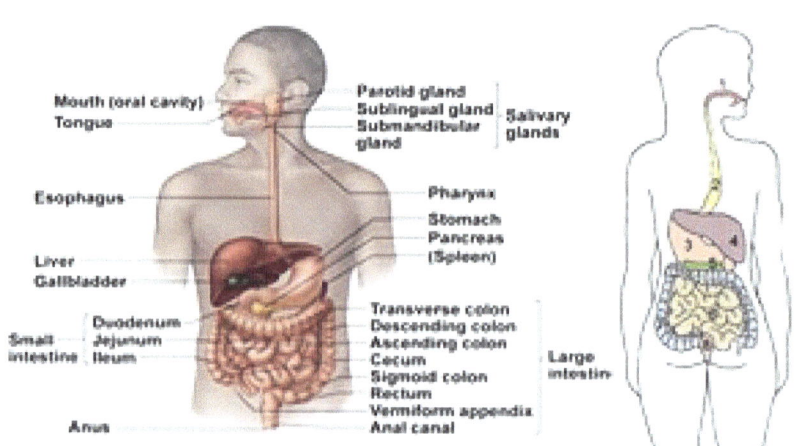

Digestive System of Male and Female

Fasting has a close relationship to the digestive system, Ramadan practically does not mean anything other than abstaining from food and drink any omission of the digestive system with the performance of his mission or his job since sunrise to sunset, and thus constitutes a fasting rest of this device for more than 12 hours during which they may pick up his breath and restoration of many of the corruptions Over the whole month.

This is a device that receives food and digest and turns and is the process of absorption of the elements useful and needed him, is responsible, then the feelings of satiety, hunger and appetite and fullness, but this machine psyche of its own reflected in various outburst of agitation and swelling, colic, and indigestion, which is also the starting point also for many of our diseases.

During Ramadan show a lot of digestive problems, a large number of patients confused in rebate in the case of fasting or their breakfast, where wary of many of the complications that may inevitably vary from disease to disease.

But the consensus of doctors is that in the fast, there is maximum benefit for the digestive system.

So everyone can afford to pay attention to the thought, for example, that fasting always improves digestion, and we have to ask ourselves: Do we not automatically refrain from eating whenever we feel that the food we ate caused us some colic and indigestion?

We feel directly and then after a while or a lot of rest and get rid of digestion disorder.

This is not only our observation we are, it is a proven fact has documented many of the doctors who tried to fast treatment, including Dr. Taner who treated indigestion accompanied him since childhood fasting and fasting only!!

He also spoke of how some doctors that fasting helps the patient to recover from the stomach through the reduction of acid secretions due to lack of food, where they can take advantage of the mucous membrane of the victim and the sufferer following the rest period equal to wellness and healing. Also does not exclude the fast reproduction of the intestine where necessary comfort in turn is the scene of continuous cleaning and disinfection of toxins , the rest of the stomach digestion and relax the intestinal absorption and the intervention of the gallbladder and pancreas in a temporary slumber but it is useful in order to improve performance and efficiency.

Therefore, the general rule is that the diseases of the digestive system do not prevent fasting in general, and that fasting does not cause diseases of the digestive system or lead to complications.

Peptic ulcer:

The erosion topical in the mucous membrane lining the wall of the stomach or duodenal, as though there are secretions of the stomach containing a strong acid and enzymes digestive but there are effective mechanisms for the protection of the wall of the stomach and intestines, so the ulcer of the digestive system is not only a reflection of the failure mechanisms of protection following or hyperthyroidism secretion of the aforementioned articles and all this happens in the following cases:

Infection: infected with the bacterium Helicobacter pylori or by the weakening of the mucous membrane of the digestive system.

Excessive handling of some of the materials and drugs that cause erosion of the membrane of the digestive system, such as derivatives of aspirin and anti-inflammatory corticosteroids and materials, in addition to some factors, such as smoking and alcoholism.

Symptoms of a patient suffering from a peptic ulcer include severe pain in the upper abdomen, which lasts for several days or weeks and dims when eating or taking antibiotics for acidity. Of course there are several complications of these ulcers, which can be summarized in: weight loss, anemia, and disruptions in the functions of the gastrointestinal tract as well as in the possibility of turning stomach ulcers to cancer,in addition to the complications of emergency, which is the occurrence of severe bleeding or erosion full and be a hole or slot perforation in the wall of the stomach or intestines, so the fear of patients with ulcers of the digestive system of the Ramadan fast merely reflects the suspicion of these complications that are serious if it happened. That has put doctors rules and conditions for the fasting patient ulcers of the digestive system, where they recommend breakfast when the patient complains of acute ulcer with symptoms of pain when hungry, as well as in the event of a severe setback when suffer from chronic ulcers, or persistent symptoms of ulcers of the digestive system with patients receiving treatment regularly, and of course the breakfast is necessary in the event of complications of stomach ulcers or when prove examination endoscopic non-healing ulcers, despite follow treatment, while fasting obligatory in patients who had recovered from ulcers of the digestive system and who have demonstrated they have the examination endoscopy scar of peptic ulcers.

Indigestion:

This is a very loose description indicating an uncomfortable situation for the digestive system.

A number of symptoms that appear after eating a meal such as nausea and abdominal gas and bloating and abdominal cramps. All of these symptoms are disappeared during Ramadan if the person committed the system to eat a good balanced and moderate.

Otherwise, overeating will lead to the aggravation of these symptoms, which can not in any way be a call to return to eating.

Diarrhea:

This leads to the loss of ample amounts of water and salts. Therefore, it requires the person to break the fast, especially if it is accompanied by fever and if it is severe during the critical phase.

Reflux to the esophagus (stomach hernia):

Means that some of the disease and digestive secretions that have the character of an acid in the stomach in order to digest the food go up from the stomach into the esophagus, which is the channel that connects the mouth, and stomach and Esophagus. If the mucous membrane of the stomach lining or protective does not affect where these juices, the esophagus lacks its lining .Therefore, these secretions flowing towards the top cause burning sensation.

This feeling is caused heartburn and reflux in particular the presence of gastric hernia, and this happens hernia particularly in people suffering from obesity and obesity, especially among women around the age of thirty. In this particular case, the patient may not have any symptoms but may suffer from heartburn and acidity, especially when the stomach is filled with food or when the person is doing too much by leaning forward or when lying on the bed, where part of the contents of the stomach back up. Doctors recommend for this group of patients to eat small meals at breakfast, take medication regularly, staying away from fatty diets, to quit smoking, to stop drinking coffee, and to combat obesity in particular.

These patients are advised to leave up to four hours between eating meals and sleeping.

But in the case of whether the patient felt uncomfortable. Ramadan burden to him or worsened symptoms breakfast he can ward off complications.

Operations that cut the stomach:

These patients, due to the lack of the remaining portion of their stomachs, may have to eat small meals and eat more frequently. Therefore, in most cases, they cannot fast.

Irritable bowel syndrome:

By this name, we mean by a group of symptoms that include abdominal cramps, bloating, diarrhea, and constipation. This is a very common disease that affects 30 percent of all people.

The doctors diagnose the disease after getting a thorough history of the situation and asking about the quality of food stimuli and psychological potential for irritation of the colon, blood tests and examinations.

Attention to nutrition is the first step in treatment. If the patient noticed that certain foods or liquids provoked symptoms, these should be avoided. The doctor often adds drugs to ease the symptoms of the disease in the patient.

IBS patients differently during Ramadan, and if the patient was aware of his world in details often take the necessary precautions during eating in Ramadan shall judge this month in good health, but may improve symptoms, especially since Ramadan is commonly an atmosphere of tranquility within the soul and calms the nerves and pushes the tension.

If the patient's illness and unknowing ignorant of its causes and gone during this month in overeating and lack of food selection. It is expected to worsen symptoms and feel more without a little fatigue and discomfort.

In general, each patient's list of banned foods is created by him or her through experience. But for all IBS patients, doctors advise them to stay away from caffeine and vegetable-producing gases like beans, cabbage, dairy products, fatty foods, and soft drinks.

Gallstones

In most cases, gallstones do not cause the appearance of any symptoms, but they are always potentially dangerous. The gallbladder stores bile juice, which is one of the secretions of the liver, to facilitate the process of digesting fats; Gallstones are often detected by a sudden sharp pain that lasts for several hours. This usually begins after eating; the pain starts on the one side and wraps around the liver to the back. It is sometimes accompanied by nausea and fever.

Women are the most vulnerable to gallstones because of the female hormone estrogen, which is also found in the pill and in HRT after menopause and gallstones pose some problems for his patients are women and men, especially when the disease is diagnosed during Ramadan through echo examination.

Faced with this situation, there are several options: If the patient does not complain of any symptoms or complications and the discovery of gallstones may have been a coincidence, he or she should continue the fast and postpone the solution to the problem of gallstones until after Eid al-Fitr.

If the symptoms are so severe that they affect the everyday life of the patient (and this is rare) or if the patient is suffering from some complications, such as chronic cholecystitis with fever, a doctor who knows how to estimate cases of urgency may initiate the treatment of that patient on the spot, forcing him or her to break the fast. In any case, observations have shown a number of doctors that the symptoms of gallstones may sometimes fade in September, allowing patients to have a lull in the surgical treatment.

Liver disease

For liver disease, doctors recommend breaking the fast in many of the cases that affect the overall health of the body, especially in advanced diseases like liver cirrhosis and liver tumors or in the case of acute viral hepatitis.

Necessary measures:

In the end, it should be noted that fasting is always a rest of the stomach; it is shrinking throughout the day in the days of fasting after eating because it has been stretched throughout the year. But our food during Ramadan should remain as it was always: balanced. Rich foods slow digestion, so you must avoid fatty foods or foods rich in sugar and not drink too much coffee, tea, training to quit smoking, etc.

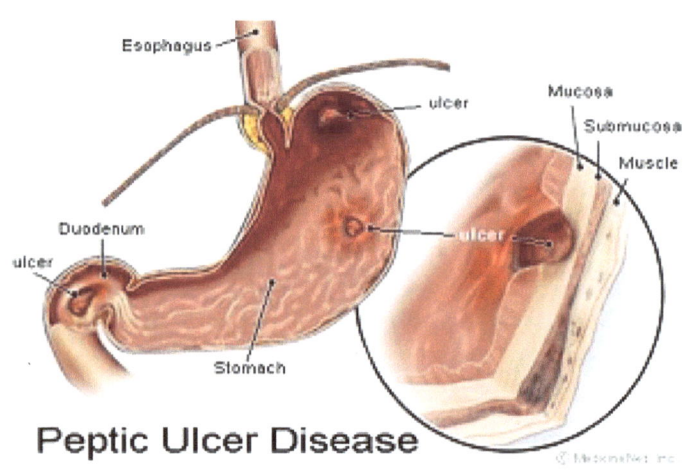

Peptic Ulcer Disease

A PEPTIC ULCER IS A HOLE IN THE GUT LINING OF THE STOMACH, DUODENUM, OR ESOPHAGUS. A PEPTIC ULCER OF THE STOMACH IS CALLED A GASTRIC ULCER; OF THE DUODENUM, A DUODENAL ULCER; AND OF THE ESOPHAGUS, AN ESOPHAGEAL ULCER. AN ULCER OCCURS WHEN THE LINING OF THESE ORGANS IS CORRODED BY THE ACIDIC DIGESTIVE JUICES WHICH ARE SECRETED BY THE STOMACH CELLS. PEPTIC ULCER DISEASE IS COMMON, AFFECTING MILLIONS OF PEOPLE YEARLY.

CHAPTER 6

Fasting and diabetic patients

In research conducted by Dr. Riad Soleimani and his colleagues at King Khalid University (1990) about the effects of Ramadan fasting on the control of diabetes, forty-seven patients with type 2 diabetes and a group of people who did not suffer from this disease were identified by body-weight protein, diabetes, and hemoglobin diabetes before Ramadan and immediately afterward. When the glycoprotein (glycosylated protein) was measured in each of the two groups, nine of the patients with diabetes were found to have had no change in weight from what it was before Ramadan (75.2 12.8) versus (75.1 12.4) kg after him, as there has been no change in the hemoglobin diabetes, (Glycosylated Hemoglobin) as it was before Ramadan (10.9 3.1) vs. (10.5 2.8) mg / ml after 100, there has been no change in the glycoprotein (Glycosylated Protein), where he was (1.19 +0.35) versus (1017 0.39), mg / 100, after the end of the Ramadan fast. In the group whose members did not suffer from diabetes, the study noted a significant reduction in weight during fasting (74.2 10.4) Kg, versus (72.5 +10.2) kg, however, there has been no significant change in hemoglobin diabetes (Glycosylated Hemoglobin).

The researchers concluded from this that the fasting month of Ramadan does not cause any significant loss in body weight, and it has no effect on the control of diabetes in disease type 2.Furthermore, Dr. (Olufonsho) and his colleagues at the faculty of medicine at King Khalid University Hospital in Riyadh (1990) distributed a questionnaire to 203 diabetic patients (89 males and 114 females) in order to assess their perceptions, attitudes, and practices during the month of Ramadan.

He has more of these (89%), fasting Ramadan, and had the lowest percentage of Siam (72%) when those who are under the age of twenty, he admitted only 12% that they are taking a greater degree of food during

Ramadan, while mention more considerable number of whom 27% said they consume deal the largest of sweets, said more than a third (37%) that their activity bodywork least in Ramadan, and the weakness of this activity was more common in those who did not fast Ramadan (61%) than among those who fasted it (35%), and showed a large number (59%) said they felt improvement in their health during the month of Ramadan, did not hesitate to hospitals in emergencies, only (5.6%) of them, while not exceeding the proportion of hospitalized because of diabetes (5%) For those who did not fast, this was less positive results, expressed as (10%) of them only for improved health, with increased emergency revisions to the hospital (15%), and wrap the cases of hospital admission (15%).

There was a widespread belief among 75% of patients that the fasting month of Ramadan led to improved health, and this was a strong feeling among patients who fasted for the month (80%) compared to those who had not fasted (26%).

The study showed that most of the diabetics prefer fasting for the month of Ramadan, and they believe that it has a positive impact on their disease.

 Some recent studies have proven that there is no pathological change or any clinical complications in patients with diabetes who fasted during Ramadan in the following components:

- Blood glucose - hemoglobin - insulin - cholesterol - and triglycerides, and body weight. Taking into account the need to take care of patients adjust their doses pharmaceutical and practicing their daily activity and in their diets, especially patients who are taking insulin.

The diabetics who are advised not to fast have been identified by the comprehensive evaluation study conducted by Dr. Soleimani and his colleagues about diabetes and fasting Ramadan in the year 1988 and are as follows:

1 - Patients who are at increased ketone bodies in the blood.

2 - Patients who suffer from a large swing and speed of change in their glucose levels.

3 - Patients who are pregnant.

4 - Children with diabetes.

5 - Diabetics who suffer from serious medical complications, such as kidney failure or angina pectoris.

6 - Diabetics who suffer from serious illnesses such as severe blood poisoning (sever sepsis) or congestive heart failure (CHF).

Allows fasting for the rest of the patients, and patients who accept medical advice and encourages fasting for obese patients of the second type who does not rely on insulin except for pregnant women and nursing mothers who have sugar steady with an increase in weight over 20% of the ideal weight.

The conclusion that most of the research suggests that the fasting month of Ramadan for diabetics safe from a health standpoint as long as there was the awareness and control of food and medicine.

Patients with type 2 can safely fast.

Lasting appetite reduction:

One of the main problems with extreme fad diets is that any weight that is lost is often quickly put back on, sometimes even with a little added extra.

This isn't the case with Ramadan. The reduction in food consumed throughout fasting causes your stomach to gradually shrink, meaning that you'll need to eat less food to feel full. If you want to get into the habit of healthy eating, then Ramadan is a great time to start.

When it's finished, your appetite will be lower than it was before, and you'll be far less likely to overindulge with your eating.

Ditch bad habits

Because you will be fasting during the day, Ramadan is the perfect time to ditch your bad habits for good.

Vices such as smoking and sugary foods should not be indulged during Ramadan and as you abstain from them, your body will gradually acclimate to their absence, until your addiction is kicked for good. It's also much easier to quit habits when you do so in a group, which should be easy to find during Ramadan.

Fasting's ability to help you cut out bad habits is so significant that the UK's National Health Service recommends it as the ideal time to ditch smoking.

Fasting is of exceptional value in the treatment of appendicitis. Recovery generally takes places within a few days to two weeks of fasting.

The advantage of fasting over surgery cases, especially those that are most severe, is seen by the fact that the mortality rate in cases of acute, gangrenous, ruptured appendicitis with peritonitis is only 1.43 percent when the operation is deferred. Immediate operations under the same conditions have provided a mortality rate of 10.64 percent (Reference: *Journal of the American Medical Association*, Dec. 5, 1936, page 1910).

Further, the average death rate in all forms of appendicitis when surgery is resorted to be 2.3 percent, with 16,000 of an average of 520,000 patients dying annually in the United States.

The efficiency of fasting in such cases is shown by the experience of Dr. Hay, who treated over four hundred patients who were afflicted with acute and chronic appendicitis.

In nineteen cases, the appendix had already ruptured.

Yet complete recovery occurred in every case, without a single failure or fatality.

In no instance was surgery resorted to. Each patient was fasted until recovery was complete.

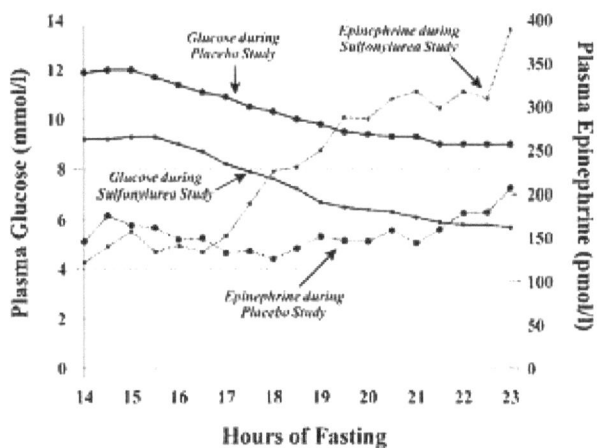

Plasma glucose (solid lines) and epinephrine (dashed lines) concentrations among fifty-two elderly type 2 diabetes patients obtained during three twenty-three-hour fasting studies after the ingestion of one week of placebo or a maximum dose (20 mg) of either glyburide or lipizide GITS. (Adapted from Burge MR, Schmitz-Fiorentino K, Fischette C, et al. "A prospective trial of risk factors for sulfonylurea-induced hypoglycemia in type 2 diabetes mellitus." *JAMA,* 1998. 279:137–143.

CHAPTER 7

The effect of fasting on heart health

The heart muscle does not diminish appreciably, deriving its sustenance from the less essential tissues. Its rate of pulsing varies greatly, rising and falling as the needs of the system demand. Studying the respiration rate, Benedict noted various minor fluctuations and arrived at the conclusion that "at least during the first two days of the fast, the pulse rate is much more liable to fluctuations than the respiration rate." That fasting benefits the heart is certain from the results obtained in functional and even in organic heart "disease" during a fast. This arises from three chief causes—namely, (1) it removes the constant stimulation of the heart; (2) it takes a heavy load off the heart and permits it to rest; (3) it purifies the blood, thus nourishing the heart with better food.

The heart that is pulsating at the rate of 80 times a minute pulsates 115,200 times in twenty-four hours. Shortly after the fast is instituted, the heart rate decreases and, while it may temporarily go much below 60 pulsations a minute, it ultimately settles at 60 beats a minute and remains there for the duration of the fast. This is 86,400 pulsations in twenty-four hours, or 28,800 fewer pulsations each day than it was doing before the fast.

This represents a decrease of twenty-five percent of the work of the heart. The saving in work is seen not merely in the reduction of the number of pulsations, but also in the vigor or force of the pulsations. It all sums up to a real vacation—a rest—for the heart. During this rest the heart repairs its damaged structures and replenishes its tissues.

As shown elsewhere, the heart muscle loses only three percent by the time death occurs from starvation. As in other essential tissues the loss of this small percent occurs after the exhaustion of the body's nutritive reserves—that is, during the starvation period. This ability of the body to nourish the heart during a prolonged fast is a sure guarantee against damage to the heart resulting from the fast.

Reviewing the chief historical examples of fasting with reference to the pulse beat, Benedict shows that in some cases the pulse remained "healthy," and in others it rose or fell. As a result of his review of these cases and of his own series of short experimental fasts, he arrived at no definite conclusions. Carrington says: "That the heart is invariably strengthened and invigorated by fasting is true beyond a doubt. I take the stand that fasting is the greatest of all strengtheners of weak hearts—being, in fact, it's only rational, physiological cure." He attributes the benefits that accrue to the heart while fasting to increased rest, a purer blood stream and absence of stimulation.

The recovery of the heart from serious impairment during a fast (I have had complete and permanent recoveries in what were thought to be incurable organic heart affections), proves that the added rest the fast affords the heart and the general renovation of the body, enable it to repair itself.

Dr. Eales says: "Instead of the heart growing weak during a fast it grows stronger every hour as the load it has been carrying is lessened." High blood pressure is invariably lowered and this removes a heavy load from the heart.

On the 15th day of his fast, friends of Dr. Eales brought him the news account of the sudden death of a man in Washington, D. C., while on a fast. The papers attributed the death to the fast, and friends of Dr. Bales warned him of heart failure. Dr. Bales replied to their warnings: "This man's death was not caused by the fast; in fact the fast lengthened his life, for if he had not been fasting he would undoubtedly have died a week or more earlier. He probably resorted to the fast to save his life, but it was too late; his light was too nearly burned out when he started. How many times do we hear of dying after a full meal, when making an after-dinner speech or sitting in their chairs and expiring! That, of course, is regular, but to die when the heart is resting and doing less work than when one is eating, when it is just worn and run down from overwork, is always attributed to fasting, if the person is fasting at the time of death."

Of the many thousands who die yearly of heart trouble, probably not more than three or four are fasting at the time of their death. In my own practice one death from "heart failure" has occurred during a fast. The patient had been considerably overweight for years, with high blood pressure, nervous troubles, glaucoma, and gave a history of diabetes. Quite naturally the failure of her heart was attributed to the fast and the fact that people in her condition die every day from "heart failure" who have not been fasting, but feeding, escapes notice. Wm. J. Bryan, who never fasted, ate a hearty meal, went to bed for an afternoon nap and never woke up. These things occur daily.

The woman was many pounds overweight at death and there could be no suggestion of starvation in this case. There were ample food reserves left in her body for another forty to fifty days of fasting.

I attribute the collapse of the heart in the above case to fear. That fear was present was manifest. That the woman had the suggestion of starvation and death dinned into her ears every day of her fast and had the suggestion intensified after the heart became affected is certain. Sudden deaths from fear, shock, etc., are not unknown or even uncommon.

"How many times," asks Dr. Eales, in discussing the effects of fear in the fast, "have we heard of sad news producing prostration or a fit of sickness; a mother's milk becoming poison during a fit of anger causing sickness to her nursing babe, and in some instances even death?"

Again he says: "I find that so long as the mind is free from worry and fear there is not a particle of danger. It is only when the subconscious mind has suggestions of weakness and fear that the body or any of its organs become weak."

Heart disease has been treated by fasting in a enormous number of cases. Fortunately the most common causes of heart trouble—narrowing of the coronary artery and formation of thrombus in this artery—are usually corrected by fasting.

As a rule the thrombus and excess fatty material lining the walls of the artery are absorbed by autolysis during the course of the fast. Other heart diseases, such as acute myocarditis, fatty overgrowth of the heart, endocarditis and ordinary pericarditis also respond very favorably to fasting. Two less common heart conditions, hemopericardium and calcified pericardium, can usually be remedied only partially when any form of help is possible to investigate whether Ramadan fasting has any effect on patients with heart disease.

METHODS:

We prospectively studied 465 outpatients with heart disease who were fasting during the month of Ramadan from October 24 to November 24, 2003. These studied subjects were from various medical centers in the Gulf region; State of Qatar, Kuwait, United Arab Emirates, and Bahrain. We performed detailed clinical assessments one month before Ramadan, during Ramadan and one month after Ramadan and analyzed predictors of outcome.

RESULTS:

Overall, the mean age was 55.9+/ 11.3 years (age range 32-72). Of the 465 patients treated, 363 (78.1%) were males and 102 (21.9%) females. Among them, 119 (25.6%) patients had congestive heart failure, 288 (62%) patients with angina, 22 (4.7%) patients with atrial fibrillation and 11 (2.4%) patients with prosthetic metallic valves. Three hundred and seventy (79%) had prior myocardial infarction (MI), 195 (17.2%) had prior coronary artery bypass surgery (CABG), and 177 (38%) had prior percutaneous coronary interventions (PCI). At the time of follow-up, we found that 91.2% could fast and only 6.7% felt worse while fasting in Ramadan. Of the studied subjects, 82.8% were compliant with cardiac medications and 68.8% were compliant with dietary instructions. We hospitalized 19 patients during Ramadan for cardiac reasons (unstable angina, worsening heart failure, MI, uncontrolled hypertension, sub therapeutic anticoagulation or arrhythmias)

CONCLUSION:

The effects of fasting during Ramadan on stable patients with cardiac diseases are minimal. Most patients with stable cardiac disease can fast.

A new study from doctors in Utah who looked at the relationship between periodic fasting and cardiovascular disease. The researchers interviewed 200 patients who were undergoing a diagnostic test called angiography, an X-ray exam of the blood vessels and heart chambers that can determine if a person has coronary heart disease.

The patients were asked if they engaged in regular fasting, and the researchers compared the answers to whether they eventually received a diagnosis of heart disease. Because about 90 percent of the patients were Mormons, a faith that encourages its members to fast for one day a month, the doctors expected to find a relatively high rate of normal fasting among the study participants.

The researchers found that people who fasted regularly had a 58 percent lower risk of coronary disease compared with those who said they didn't fast, according to the report presented at the American College of Cardiology conference in New Orleans this week.

The study showed only an association between fasting and better heart health, which means it's possible that fasting may not have a direct effect but might just be more common among people who are healthier to begin with. Devout Mormons, for instance, abstain from alcohol, smoking and caffeine, which are all factors that could affect heart health.

But the researchers say the findings are significant because they affirm the results of an earlier, larger study, published in 2008 in *The American Journal of Cardiology*, which found a similar association between fasting and heart disease among 448 patients.

"The first study we did was not a chance finding," said Dr. Benjamin D. Horne, director of cardiovascular and genetic epidemiology for Intermountain, a health services and managed care firm in Salt Lake City.

"We were able to replicate the findings and show that people who fast routinely have a lower prevalence of coronary disease."

The downside of the study is that it didn't ask for specific details on the type and duration of fasting among the patients. However, preliminary interviews suggest that the most common form of fasting involved a monthly ritual of abstaining from all food and drinking only water for 24 hours.

A second, smaller study conducted by the same research team suggests that the effects of fasting aren't just about having an overall healthy lifestyle, but that abstaining from food on a regular basis leads to metabolic changes that are good for the heart.

For that research, also presented at the New Orleans conference, 30 patients were asked to fast for 24 hours with water only. The scientists used blood tests before and after the fasting period to look at a number of different metabolic markers. Among other changes, they found that levels of human growth hormone, or HGH, surged after fasting — increasing 20 times in men and 13 times in women. The hormone is released by the body in times of starvation to protect lean muscle mass and trigger the body to start burning fat stores.

"There is a lot more to be done to fill in the research on the biological mechanism," Dr. Horne said. "But what it does suggest is that fasting is not a marker for other healthy lifestyle behaviors. It appears to be that fasting is causing some significant stress, and the body responds to that by some protective mechanisms that potentially have a beneficial long-term effect on risk of chronic disease."

Dr. Horne noted that patients shouldn't take up fasting without discussing it first with their doctor. Any fast should include water because dehydration can raise risk for stroke. He said the group was planning additional research into the potential health effects of regular fasting.

Research cardiologists at the Intermountain Medical Center Heart Institute are reporting that fasting not only lowers one's risk of coronary artery disease and diabetes, but also causes significant changes in a person's blood cholesterol levels. Both diabetes and elevated cholesterol are known risk factors for coronary heart disease.

The discovery expands upon a 2007 Intermountain Healthcare study that revealed an association between fasting and reduced risk of coronary heart disease, the leading cause of death among men and women in America. In the new research, fasting was also found to reduce other cardiac risk factors, such as triglycerides, weight, and blood sugar levels.

The findings were presented on April 3, at the annual scientific sessions of the American College of Cardiology in New Orleans.

"These new findings demonstrate that our original discovery was not a chance event," says Dr. Benjamin D. Horne, PhD, MPH, director of cardiovascular and genetic epidemiology at the Intermountain Medical Center Heart Institute, and the study's principal investigator. "The confirmation among a new set of patients that fasting is associated with lower risk of these common diseases raises new questions about how fasting itself reduces risk or if it merely indicates a healthy lifestyle."

Unlike the earlier study by the team, this new research recorded reactions in the body's biological mechanisms during the fasting period. The participants' low-density lipoprotein cholesterol (LDL-C, the "bad" cholesterol) and high-density lipoprotein cholesterol (HDL-C, the "good" cholesterol) both increased (by 14 percent and 6 percent, respectively) raising their total cholesterol—and catching the researchers by surprise.

"Fasting causes hunger or stress. In response, the body releases more cholesterol, allowing it to utilize fat as a source of fuel, instead of glucose. This decreases the number of fat cells in the body," says Dr. Horne. "This is important because the fewer fat cells a body has, the less likely it will experience insulin resistance, or diabetes."

This recent study also confirmed earlier findings about the effects of fasting on human growth hormone (HGH), a metabolic protein. HGH works to protect lean muscle and metabolic balance, a response triggered and accelerated by fasting. During the 24-hour fasting periods, HGH increased an average of 1,300 percent in women, and nearly 2,000 percent in men.

In this most recent trial, researchers conducted two fasting studies of over 200 individuals—both patients and healthy volunteers—who were recruited at Intermountain Medical Center. A second 2011 clinical trial followed another 30 patients who drank only water and ate nothing else for 24 hours. They were also monitored while eating a healthy diet during an additional 24-hour period. Blood tests and physical measurements were taken from all to evaluate cardiac risk factors, markers of metabolic risk, and other general health parameters.

While the results were surprising to researchers, it's not time to start a fasting diet just yet. It will take more studies like these to fully determine the body's reaction to fasting and its effect on human health. Dr. Horne believes that fasting could one day be prescribed as a treatment for preventing diabetes and coronary heart disease.

To help achieve the goal of expanded research, the Deseret Foundation (which funded the previous fasting studies) recently approved a new grant to evaluate many more metabolic factors in the blood using stored samples from the recent fasting clinical trial. The researchers will also include an additional clinical trial of fasting among patients who have been diagnosed with coronary heart disease.

"We are very grateful for the financial support from the Deseret Foundation. The organization and its donors have made these groundbreaking studies of fasting possible," added Dr. Horne.

Members of the Intermountain Medical Center Heart Institute research team included Dr. Horne, Jeffrey L. Anderson, MD, John F. Carlquist, PhD, J. Brent Muhlestein, MD, Donald L. Lappé, MD, Heidi T. May, PhD, MSPH, Boudi Kfoury, MD, Oxana Galenko, PhD, Amy R. Butler, Dylan P. Nelson, Kimberly D. Brunisholz, Tami L. Bair, and Samin Panahi.

Effect of fasting on blood pressure:

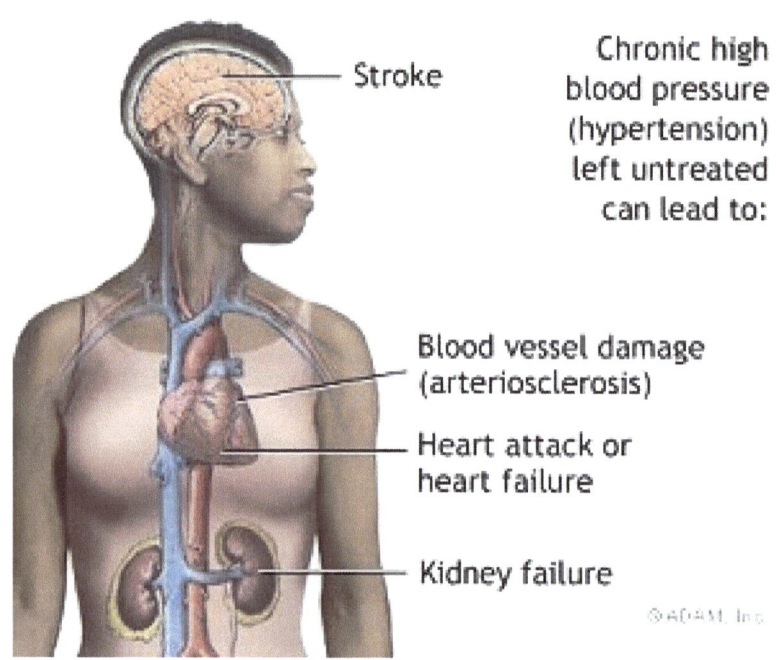

Hypertension is a disorder characterized by chronically high blood pressure. It must be monitored, treated and controlled by medication, lifestyle changes, or a combination of both.

Fasting is without doubt the most rapid and efficient method of remedying high blood pressure. Indeed, hundreds of consecutive patients have been treated for this condition without a single complete failure.

Even patients who have failed to respond to all of the customary treatment of high blood pressure do respond to fasting.

Shelton has reported one case in which a systolic pressure of 295 was brought down to 115 during three weeks of fasting. And the cures in these cases tend to be lasting.

If the blood pressure falls below normal during the fast, it will rise to normal later, but actual hypertension does not redevelop so long as good nutritional habits are maintained after the fast.

Heart disease has been treated by fasting in a enormous number of cases. Fortunately the most common causes of heart trouble—narrowing of the coronary artery and formation of thrombus in this artery—are usually corrected by fasting.

As a rule the thrombus and excess fatty material lining the walls of the artery are absorbed by autolysis during the course of the fast.

Other heart diseases, such as acute myocarditis, fatty overgrowth of the heart, endocarditis and ordinary pericarditis also respond very favorably to fasting. Two less common heart conditions, hem pericardium and calcified pericardium, can usually be remedied only partially when any form of help is possible.

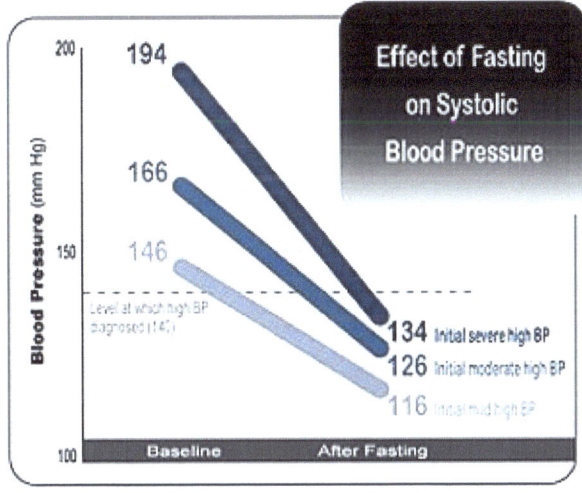

Effect of fasting on blood clotting:

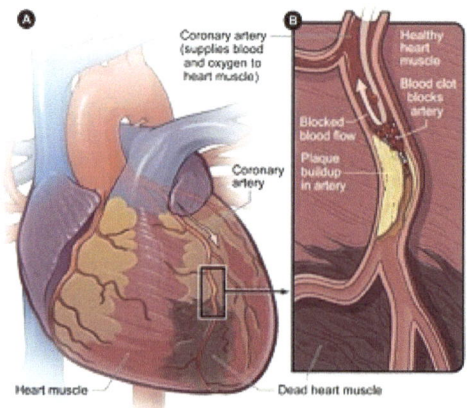

Figure A is an overview of a heart and coronary artery showing damage (dead heart muscle) caused by a heart attack. Figure B is a cross-section of the coronary artery with plaque buildup and a blood clot resulting from plaque rupture.

Besides actually lowering blood pressure, fasting removes and softens the cholesterol plaque that lines the blood vessels. Surgery, atherectomy, and angioplasty, the invasive approaches to coronary artery disease, will always remain ineffective at significantly extending life. This is because these procedures address only the localized blockage. This small area of diseased blood vessel, though it may be the source of chest pain, will not necessarily be the area that causes death should a person suffer a fatal heart attack. Concentrating on a localized area of coronary artery narrowing in a body full of vessels with diffuse atherosclerotic plaque is like trying to save a patient with advanced metastatic cancer by removing one surgically accessible mass.

"Fasting thins the blood and prevents blood clots, or thrombi. Platelets do not clot as easily during fasting, and the ability of the red blood cells to clump together is diminished. Therefore, the fast quickly lowers an individual's risk of a heart attack.

"The potential of a total fast (water only) to induce biochemical changes within the body that prevent formation of a thrombus has been well documented. (Muliar LA, Mishchenko VP, Loban GA, Goncharenko LL, Bobyrev VN. Effect of complete fasting on the coagulative and antioxidative properties of blood. Voprosy Pitaniya 1984; 4:20–23.) In one such study a fast was undertaken by 22 healthy volunteers. The ability of their blood to clot and form a thrombus under fasting conditions was extensively analyzed. Fasting was discovered to lead to the reduction of blood plasma and red cell coagulation, deterioration of platelet aggregation, a rise of the oxidized hemoglobin content, and an increase in red cell resistance to peroxide hemolysis. In short, fasting lowers the risk of intravascular coagulation and thrombus formation.

"Other studies have shown that after 36 hours of fasting there is a significant increase in the fibrinolytic activity of the blood. Fibrinolysis is the breakdown of clots. This activity continues for 24 hours after the fast is terminated (Miettinen M. Effect of fasting on fibrinolysis and blood coagulation. Amer J Cardiol 1962; 10:532–534. Menon IS. Fasting and non-fasting fibrinolytic activity. Lab Prac 1967; 16:469–470."

It was thought that the loss relative to body fluids, low heart rate, and increased stress during fasting, have a negative impact on the control blood clots, it the one of the most dangerous diseases, has proven to be fasting. Muslim does not affect that in patients taking specific doses of treatment.

A study was conducted by Dr. Jalal Saaour, professor of internal medicine at King Faisal Specialist Hospital (1990), in search of the effect of fasting on heart patients who are taking antiretroviral treatment for blood clots. In a written a summary of his research, Dr. Saaour said:

The majority of muslims accepts the fasting month of Ramadan every year, and the consequent fasting occurrence of significant changes in physical activity and sleep patterns, as well as the changing times to eat and drink, and kind, and therefore it is possible to affect fasting negative impact on the control to prevent clotting of during the relative loss of body fluids, low cardiac output, increased stress, and blood viscosity, as well as changes to occur in the absorption and metabolism of medicines.

In the period between 1981 to 1985 were examined a total of 289 patients in the clinic to prevent blood clotting King Faisal Specialist Hospital, receiving 247 patients, of whom antiretroviral treatment of a blood clot, due to the condition of the heart they have, and 42 due to the clot deep in the veins, with pulmonary embolism or without it.

In the treatment period (4 years), fasted for 106 of these patients, a total of 309 months Ramadan, did not fast number 183 of them, a total of 594 months.

It was observed that the incidence of thromboembolic complications and bleeding similar in the two groups, and the average dose of warfarin 4 needed to bring the best effect to prevent clotting in the two groups during the month of Ramadan identical: 5. 6 +1.2 7.6 mg versus 2.2 mg.

Since 1986, we advise our patients who are taking treatment against thrombosis by mouth, that there is no harm from their fast month of Ramadan, and has during this period, 277 patients have valves, alternative fasting total of 1054 months, and did not appear on any of them in this time complications of obstructive thromboembolic.

The possible consequences of the long intermittent fasting schedule during Ramadan (one month of food and water intake limited to night hours, a practice that is followed by the majority of the Muslims worldwide) on certain biochemical constituents or coagulation variables have not been extensively documented.

Patients and Methods: During the month of Ramadan and two months after, we monitored the concentration of different plasma lipoproteins, lipoprotein (a) [Lp (a)], apoproteins A1 and B, fibrinogen, factor VII activity and some selected hematological factors in 50 healthy subjects who were employees of institutes related to the Isfahan University of Medical Sciences and aged between 30 and 45 years.

The effect of fasting in Ramadan on the relationship between biochemical and coagulation variables was also investigated.

Results: The values of apoprotein B, Lp(a) and low-density lipoprotein cholesterol (LDL-C)/high-density lipoprotein cholesterol (HDL-C) ratio were significantly decreased during Ramadan ($P<0.05$), while total cholesterol (Tot-C), triglycerides (TG), LDL-C, HDL-C and fasting blood glucose did not change during that month.

Among coagulation and hematological factors, fibrinogen level and factor VII activity were significantly decreased during the month ($P<0.05$). Results also indicated a significant positive association between fibrinogen level and LP (a), factor VII activity and Tot-C, LDL-C, TG and Apo B during Ramadan.

Conclusion: Our findings contribute to a better understanding of previous reports, as the metabolic and coagulation changes that are considered as atherosclerosis risk factors are counterbalanced during Ramadan.

Ann Saudi Med 2000; 20(5-6):377-381.

Key Words: Ramadan, fasting, blood lipids, fibrinogen, factor VII.

During the holy month of Ramadan (the ninth lunar month of the Muslim year), it is obligatory for all adult Muslims to abstain from food, drink and smoking each day from dawn to sunset.

Usually, the quality of food and eating patterns changes to the consumption of more carbohydrates and sweet foods, mainly in the form of two large meals at dawn and sunset.

Several studies have reported on the physiological effects of Ramadan, especially concerning changes in blood pressure, lipids, apoproteins, fasting blood sugar (FBS), hormones and other biochemical parameters Other reports have attempted to study the effect of fasting during that month on the values of certain hemostatic, fibrinolytic, platelet aggregation and coagulation factors, however, the association between biochemical factors such as apoproteins, lipoprotein (a) [Lp(a)] and coagulation factors such as fibrinogen or factor VII, an important interrelationship between some atherosclerotic risk factors that have been previously reported, have not yet been studied during the month of Ramadan.

Patients and Methods:

Fifty adult employees of institutes related to Isfahan University of Medical Sciences were identified by simple random sampling.

The study was conducted on the 26th day of the month and repeated two months later.

The subjects (22 males and 28 females) were aged between 30 and 45 years and were fasting for the whole month.

They were found to be healthy on general medical examination and none was receiving any medication affecting the studied parameters.

Histories were taken and some anthropometric variables were identified.

Blood pressure was measured according to the technique described by WHO. Blood samples were taken on the 26th day of Ramadan at 4 p.m., then two months later, after 12 hours of fasting.

All blood samples were sent to the Central Laboratory of Isfahan Cardiovascular Research Center. Hematological parameters were estimated on fresh blood using Cell Counter AL820. Clotting time (CT) and bleeding time (BT) were measured using Lee White method.

Prothrombin time (PT) and partial thromboplastin time (PTT) were estimated using turbidimetric methods by Neoplastin Ciplus and C.K. Prest kits, respectively.

Fibrinogen was measured by turbidimetric method using coagulometer Cascade M4 and Fibri-Prest Automate kits.

Plasma factor VII activity (%) was assessed with a one stage test plasma was added to plasma deficient in assay.

Factor VII, and the clotting time was measured, then factor VII activity was calculated by reference to a standard graph produced by testing dilution of normal human plasma.

The blood samples were also analyzed for FBS, plasma triglycerides (TG), total cholesterol (Tot-C) and high-density lipoprotein (HDL-C) by enzymatic method using Merck reagent kits and Elan 2000 autoanalyser .LDL-C was calculated by the Friedewald formula18: low-density lipoprotein (LDL-C)=Tot-C-(TG/5+HDL-C).

Lipoprotein (a) [Lp (a)] was measured by an ELISA method using Macro Lp(a) kits.

A turbidimetric immunoassay was used for determining Apo lipoproteins A1 and B by kits from Sigma.

Reference samples were created at the start of the study and included in each day's analysis to check laboratory variation.

For quality control, Isfahan Cardiovascular Research Center Laboratory meets the criteria of the central standard laboratory of the Ministry of Health in Iran. Also the samples for blood lipids were sent to the Central Laboratory, St. Rafacl University, Department of Epidemiology, Belgium, under different numbers unknown to the laboratory, and the highly significant correlation between the results from the two laboratories allowed us to use the results for international comparison.

All calculations were done using the SPSS-V6 statistical software package (the system for statistics) for analysis of the data.

All data were expressed as mean±SD. Comparisons between means observed during and after Ramadan was tested using paired t-test.

The data within each phase were also examined using Pearson's correlation analysis to find the relationship between the studied variables.

Coagulation and hemostatic factors were used as dependent variables and biochemical parameters were used as the independent ones.

All differences were considered significant at P<0.05.

Results: FBS, Tot-C, LDL-C, HDL-C, Tot-C/HDL-C ratio, TG and Apo A1 showed no significant changes during Ramadan or two months later (Table 1), however, the values of Lp(a), Apo B and LDL-C/HDL-C ratio were significantly decreased during fasting in Ramadan (P<0.05) (Table 1). Although Apo A1 was increased during Ramadan, this change was not significant (P>0.05).

CHAPTER 8

The effect of fasting on the brain and nervous system

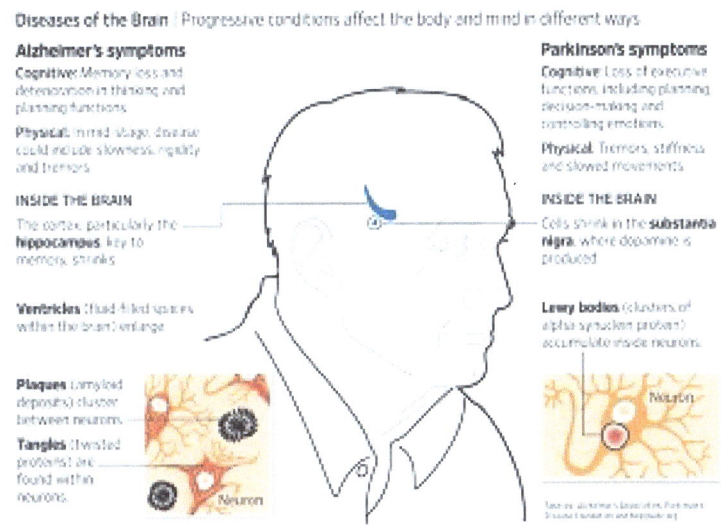

Many scientists have sought to explain the underlying mechanism by which fasting therapy corrects abnormal and unbalanced psycho-physiological systems, and restores health so efficiently. Its stabilizing effects on the nervous system have been measured electrically through brain wave recordings and its effects on the endocrine glands have been traced bio-chemically. Both sets of findings tend to confirm that fasting allows the autonomic systems of the body to function at a relaxed baseline level, free from the erratic and disruptive influences of the nervous system and hormones.

Suzuki et al. in 1976 studied changes in the brain waves from 262 fasting patients and noted a slowing and synchronization of alpha waves, together with an increased incidence of theta waves. 1) These observations are descriptive of a more relaxed and introspective state of awareness, which is less neurotically preoccupied with the superficial and transitory patterns of thought that characterize the normal waking state. Similar brain wave alterations were recorded in Zen meditators by Kasamatsu and Hirai (1966) 2) and by Banquet (1973) in subjects practicing japa yoga. 3 This suggests that fasting and meditation exert similar psycho-physiological influences on the brain and nervous system, perhaps healing psychosomatic complaints and maintaining optimal health and well-being by a single standard mechanism.

The significant slowing of brain waves suggests that fasting induces a transient slowing down of the central nervous system. It seems plausible that more complex changes in the autonomic nerves and endocrine glands may then occur. An over active autonomic nervous system, which constantly relays abnormal mental and psychic stresses into the physiological systems, produces many psychosomatic symptoms and disease states, Through fasting and meditation these stresses are removed, allowing the mechanisms responsible for blood pressure, respiratory and cardiac rate, gastrointestinal secretion and motility, etc. to revert spontaneously to a more natural level of functioning.

In Suzuki's study, this brain wave phenomenon disappeared upon termination of fasting therapy, and peak EEG frequency and wave configuration returned to a pattern strikingly similar to pre-fasting discharge patterns. However, in a more recent Japanese study of 380 fasting patients 4), where the EEG analysis was more sophisticated, peak rate decreased significantly at the end of the fasting period, suggesting that a stable new physiological state is created in the post-fasting period. In addition, the overload of fast beta waves observed in the pre-fasting period decreased in the fasting period, and did not reappear again in the same fashion after the recovery phase. As these faster waves have been associated with anxiety, tension, neuroticism and irritation, their disappearance on EEG may be an objective indication that fasting either partially or wholly eases these symptoms permanently.

Recently, the metabolic changes induced by fasting have also been investigated. The normal metabolic fuel of the brain is glucose, released into the bloodstream from the digestion of dietary carbohydrates and sugars. The research of G.F. Cahill of Joslin Research Laboratory, Harvard Medical School, USA (1966–1969), revealed that this situation changes dramatically during fasting. As the fast proceeds, the body's stores of carbohydrates in the liver are rapidly exhausted, and the brain's requirements for glucose, its sole fuel, must then be met by non-carbohydrate sources. The new source is the ketone body, derived from the hydrolysis of fat stored in the body's adipose tissues.

It appears that the brain's switch from starch to ketone nutrition works as a potent stressor upon the brain cells, and temporarily places all biological mechanisms in a stress state. This may activate the natural healing power inherent in the human body, thereby bringing about homeostasis, and a return to healthy function.

As for the headaches during fasting:

For patients with chronic migraines in the holy month of Ramadan, there are some cases where this was improved by fasting, especially if they were smokers. Ramadan month is a great opportunity to quit smoking once and for all.

In cases where the patient re-migraine attacks advising him to start treatment on dinner food (suhoor).

For those who suffer from headaches during fasting, the reason is diet and hunger in Ramadan when some fasting is hunger Psychological hungers is not contagious and therefore notes that fasting during the day combines the delicious and desirable. Himself and his greed hungry from food and put it on the breakfast table and after breakfast does not find it eat only a part of this amóunt, and this denotes the feeling of hunger is hunger myself more than hunger actual terms that the body needs very little food to fill the gap and must be in control of this hunger Psychological where we are waste a lot of the foods we claimed to provide to the actual need.

Stalking fasting headache not only during fasting but approximately one hour after breakfast and the reason for this is due to the disruption of meals at breakfast and in order to be healthy and balanced food in quantity and quality must take into account the following:

1 - The breakfast starts drinking it warm to alert juicers gastrointestinal tract because then excreted few sugars or starches to feed the brain, which needs to prices and then a few hours later start fasting food ordinary and not so frequently does not get lazy or headaches.

2 - Fault to begin fasting fluids frozen because the ice cream infect the stomach and intestines semi temporary paralysis leads to a sense of bloating, pain and lack of secretion of digestive juices and thus not digest and lengthening the duration of the food in the stomach leads to headache, fatigue, and the best doctors to follow system starts right where his breakfast coffee and then pass on prayer and rest an hour or two and then eating the main meal without overeating.

3 - Must contain all the food breakfast on the amount of vegetables and fruit to stimulate the nervous system in the brain is fasting during the day and not feeling headache and laziness.

4 - The bad habits of some fasts are sleep and inactivity and obesity, which is also the most dangerous diseases of this age because of the lack of burning what to eat at dinner (suhoor).

There are some tips that we provide to our patients, some of the brain, nerves, whose illness prevents them from fasting:

1 - Patients who have suffered a previous stroke and brain due to lack of repeat clots.

2 - Seniors (over sixty or seventy) has happened to them early warning of a heart stroke incidence.

3 - Some brain tumors.

4 - Epilepsy patients who are taking continuous treatment.

Peripheral vascular disease:

Treatment of fasting, a number of diseases caused by obesity: as a disease, atherosclerosis, and blood pressure, and certain heart diseases. It also helps in the treatment of some diseases of the peripheral circulation, there are many diseases affecting peripheral vascular, and which seem to be related to an active sympathetic nervous system (sympathetic) excess at the ends of arteries (Arterioles), and the disease is (Raynaud's Disease) one of these diseases, where constrict the muscles of the walls of the arteries minute Systole self-severe, causing intense pain, and attack these pains when exposed to cold or stress, even if the condition persists for several years may lead to the loss of the Parties, and treatment of this disease prevents exposure to the cold as much as possible, and avoid smoking, and given Some medications the patient to extend of blood vessels, also excised sympathetic nerve supplying the local parties, and avoid exposure to neurological and psychological pressure.

There is another similar disease (Burger's Disease), which affects the arteries and veins. Smoking activates the disease and is exacerbated by, and when the smoking ban improves patient improved markedly, some patients may need to eradicate the sympathetic nerve (sympathetic) nutritious parties, and sometimes the patient needs to the amputation of limbs if continued smoking.

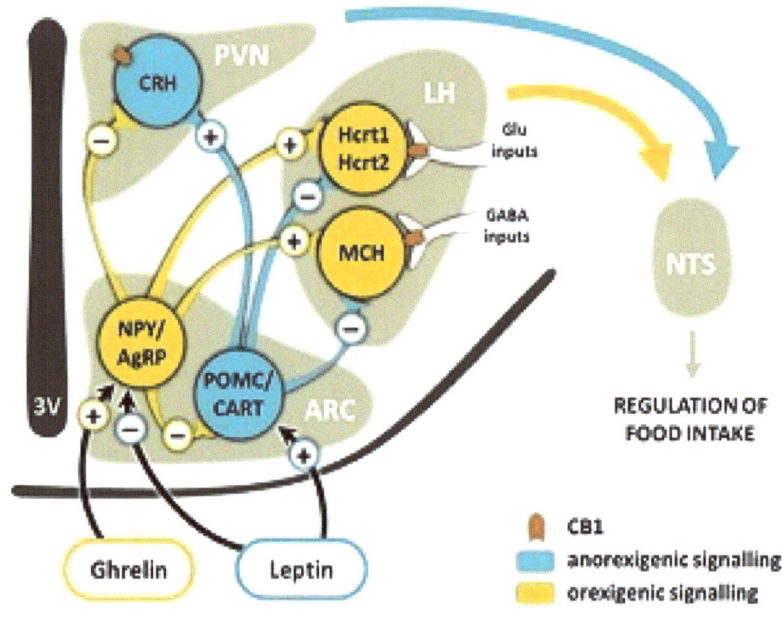

Schematic representation of the main brain pathways involved in the homeostatic control of food intake.

Fasting Boosts Neuronal Autophagy:

Autophagy, or "self-eating," is the process by which cells recycle waste material, down regulate wasteful processes, and repair themselves. Brain health is highly dependent on neuronal autophagy. In fact, a recent paper shows that deletion of an "essential autophagy gene" in the hypothalamic neurons of fetal mice resulted in metabolic derangement (more body fat, reduced glucose tolerance) and impaired neuronal development. Another study shows that disruption of neuronal autophagy induces neurodegeneration. Simply put, without the process of autophagy, brains neither develop properly nor function the way they should.

Fasting Increases Levels of Brain-Derived Neurotrophic Factor (BDNF):

BDNF is a protein that interacts with neurons in the hippocampus, cortex, and basal forebrain (the parts of the brain that regulate memory, learning, and higher cognitive function – uniquely human stuff). It helps existing neurons survive while spurring the growth of new neurons (neurogenesis) and the development of synapses (lines of communication between neurons). Low levels of BDNF are linked to Alzheimer's, and supplementary BDNF prevents neuronal death, memory loss, and cognitive impairment in an animal model of Alzheimer's disease.

Fasting Increases Production of Ketones:

The Four Phases of Fasting

Ketone bodies like hydroxybutyrate are famously neuroprotective, and fasting often induces ketosis.

Increased autophagy and BDNF and ketones from fasting sounds awesome, but do they manifest as actual benefits to neurological health? Let's see what the research says.

No discussion of fasting and neurological health research is complete (or can even be initiated) without including Mark Mattson. Mattson, chief neuroscientist at the National Institute on Aging, has been releasing paper after paper on the neurological effects of intermittent fasting for the past dozen years, and he's amassed an impressive body of work that suggests IF can induce neurogenesis and protect against brain injury and disease. In the following sections, I'll discuss the evidence – from Mattson and other researchers – for the beneficial effects of fasting on neurological health across a spectrum of conditions.

Stroke:

The most common type of strokes are ischemic strokes (composing about 88% of all strokes)—cerebrovascular events in which a blood vessel that supplies blood to the brain is blocked by a clot. Without blood, the brain can't get oxygen or nutrients, and (often permanent) brain damage can occur. In an animal model of ischemic stroke, fasting up regulated BDNF and other neuroprotective proteins, reduced mortality and inflammation, and increased cognitive health and function. However, it's worth noting that fasting was most effective against stroke in young animals, who enjoyed a four-fold increase in neuroprotective and neurogenerative BDNF. Middle aged mice saw a two-fold increase in BDNF, while older mice saw no increase. Post-stroke cognitive function had a similar relationship to age and feeding status; young and middle-aged fasted mice retained far more than old mice and fed mice. Fasted mice displayed lower levels of inflammatory cytokines, but this effect was also modulated by age. Overall, fasting increased neuroprotective proteins and decreased inflammatory cytokines in young and middle-aged mice, thereby reducing the brain damage incurred by stroke.

Brain Trauma:

Research indicates that fasting is also effective against physical trauma to the brain. It's not that fasting somehow physically repels impending trauma by generating a magical ketone-powered force field; it's that fasting reduces the oxidative stress, mitochondrial dysfunction, and cognitive decline that typically result from brain trauma. Employing one of these contraptions, researchers induced a "controlled cortical impact" on fasting rats and found that a 24-hour fast (but not a 48-hour fast) was neuroprotective. Perhaps the reduced appetite that commonly accompanies a concussion is a protective mechanism rather than an annoying side effect?

Cervical Spine Injury:

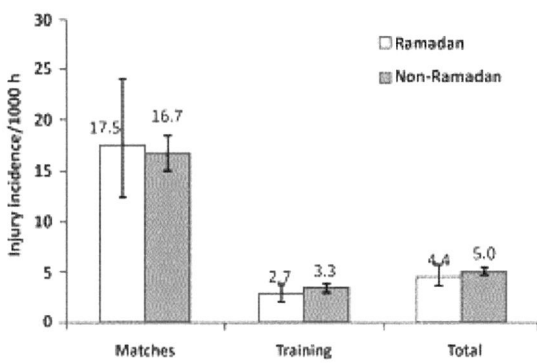

Injury incidence with upper 95% CI during training

"Every other day" fasting was neuroprotective following an injury to a rat's cervical spine. Despite extensive trauma, fasted rats improved gait pattern, vertical exploration, and forelimb function (all heavily dependent on brain function). Neuronal integrity was preserved, cortical lesion volume was reduced, and corticospinal axon (nerve fiber) sprouting increased. The same team performed a similar study on mice suffering from a spinal cord injury, but had very different results; every other day fasting failed to confer any neuroprotective or functional benefits to the injured mice whatsoever. How can we reconcile these apparently contradictory findings? Well, in the rats who experienced neuroprotection, fasting increased ketone production by 2 or 3 fold. The fasting mice never reached ketosis. Ketosis was key.

Alzheimer's disease:

In a mouse model of Alzheimer's disease, both intermittent fasting and 40% (!) calorie restrictions conferred cognitive and behavioral benefits when compared to mice on the control diet. IF and CR mice showed higher levels of exploratory behavior, and, when placed in a Morris water maze, found the escape platform sooner than the control mice. However, only IF mice showed evidence of protection against synaptic pathology—a hallmark of the disease.

Huntington's disease:

Huntington's disease is also characterized by a depletion in BDNF levels. In a rat model of the disease, intermittent fasting normalized BDNF levels, while regular feeding kept them small. Fasting rats lived longer and even enjoyed better glucose tolerance than ad libitum fed rats. By all accounts, fasting slowed progression of Huntington's disease.

Age-Related Cognitive Decline:

We've all had a grandmother who called us by our sibling's name, or a grandpa who forgot to unwrap the Worther's Original before popping it into his mouth—these are the innocent, simple, quaint, seemingly unavoidable declines in cognition that accompany the aging process. Well, maybe they aren't unavoidable. Although most of the research focuses on neurological trauma and disease, there's evidence that intermittent fasting is right for underlying age-related cognitive decline. I find it interesting that this was "late-onset" intermittent fasting; meaning elderly rats who began fasting only after showing signs of decline still wrought cognitive benefits. Contrast that with the stroke study in which more aged rodents saw almost no benefit from fasting and a picture emerges: as long as they're not trying to counter a debilitating event, like ischemic stroke or trauma, older brains can also expect to benefit from fasting.

Depression:

Depression has long been associated with lower BDNF levels as a prognostic of the disease, but it's only recently that researchers are entertaining the possibility that low BDNF and depression could be causally related. And indeed – antidepressants actually increase BDNF signaling and synthesis in the hippocampus (the part of the brain where depression "happens"). Could fasting help with depression via up regulation of BDNF and promotion of neurogenesis? Perhaps, I'd say it's worth a shot, especially since skipping a few meals doesn't require a prescription.

Obviously, since these are mostly rodent studies, and hard-and-fast peer-reviewed evidence of the neuroprotective and neurogenerative effects of fasting in humans doesn't exist yet, we're only speculating. But I'd argue they are plausible speculations worth pursuing. The mechanisms are there. A speculation about IF's other health effects—to general health and cancer and longevity and fat loss—are being borne out by human research. Both the risk and barrier to entry are small. And it makes sense in light of our evolutionary history as hunter-gatherers. In a recent interview, Mattson even couches the neuroprotective effects of fasting in evolutionary terms, noting that during pre-agricultural times of scarcity, people "whose brains responded best—who remembered where promising sources could be found or recalled how to avoid predators—would have been the ones who got the food" and lived to pass on their genes.

The Difference between Fasting and Anorexia:

Fasting is total abstinence from food for a relatively short period of time determined by natural conditions. The motivation for fasting is not weight-loss but improved health. Fasting involves an application of millennia-old principles to attain better health (or in some cases a heightened mental and spiritual state). During fasting, hunger is naturally absent and returns when the fast ends. The results of fasting are all active: improved health and longevity and removal of toxic and morbid matter from the body. Energy and outlook are improved.

Anorexia seems to stem not from the desire to be healthy but gaunt, an erroneous idea promulgated by the movie industry. In anorexia, an insufficient amount of food is eaten over an extended period, causing a lack of protein, vitamins, minerals, essential fatty acids, and other essential nutrients. There is a state of mind that hypnotically blots out hunger, which results in malnutrition (a state that has never been recorded to occur during fasting). Anorexia ends from outside pressure, forced feeding, or death from malnutrition.

The dreaded disease, multiple sclerosis:

Multiple sclerosis has been treated successfully with fasting. Dr. Shelton states that "much progress may be expected in a great number" of late cases of this disease, even though recovery is not entirely complete. Dr. Richard Geithner, of the Blaubeuren Sanatorium in Germany, reported that three multiple sclerosis patients "who agreed to the fasting-cure were free of paralysis after 18 to 21 days of fasting." One of these patients had a new episode of paralysis after the fast, which, in turn, was cured by another fast of 14 days. During the following three years of observation, there was no recurrence of paralysis.

Dr. Alsaker stated that "It is a revelation to some persons who fast how precisely the mind can function." This being true, it might be expected that various forms of insanity would be helped by fasting. Widespread experience by many physicians has shown that fasting is not only valuable in caring for the insane patient but that it frequently succeeds where all other forms of treatment have failed. Fasting can not only be applied in promoting absorption of brain tumors and improving the physical condition of the brain and nervous system; it also has been used successfully in treating mental aberrations which were thought to have purely emotional causes.

Of those fasting practitioners who have cared for mental patients, Dr. Hay had some of the most notable experiences. He applied the absolute fast and partial fast, along with proper nutrition, and he reported excellent results in the majority of cases. Of seventeen cases of dementia praecox brought to Dr. Hay, five cases were unmanageable without restraint but all others were carefully treated and "made splendid comebacks" to a high grade of mental health. Dr. Hay described one mental patient who "was wholly irrational, could not even answer questions having both amnesic and ataxic aphasia, cried continually, and required a special nurse to restrain her from throwing herself out of the window." Yet after ten days of partial fasting, utilizing only the extracted juices of fruits and vegetables, followed by 20 days of controlled diet, the patient returned to her home "as sane as she had ever been before in her life, and a very bright young woman."

CHAPTER 9

The effect of fasting on the endocrine glands

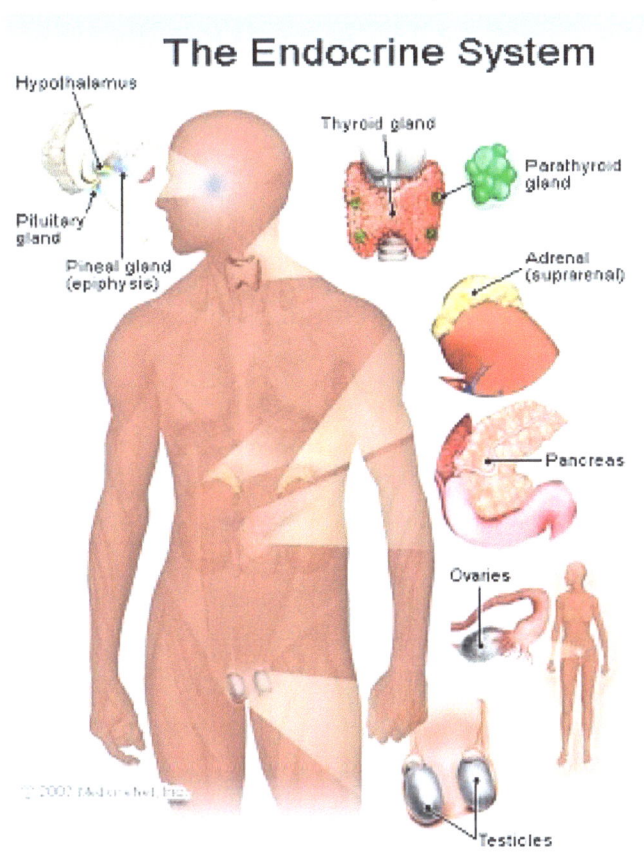

Disordered function of the network of endocrine glands, with their secretion of abnormal and ill-timed quantities of hormones into the bloodstream, is a potent cause of physiological disruption. In addition, abnormal blood concentrations of gonadal, pituitary, adrenal and thyroid hormones are now recognized to be a major determinant of unhealthy emotional and psychological states, profoundly affecting mental health and wellbeing.

Endocrinologists are able to assess the function of the hypothalamus-pituitary-adrenal axis of glands by measuring the levels of hormone by products found in the urine and blood. In the 1979 Tohoku study, this analysis indicated that the activity of the hypothalamus-pituitary-adrenal axis declines during fasting. This state is very similar to that which occurs immediately after the endocrine glands have been activated by a stress situation. At that time, after the initial burst of secretion, there is a stable or refractory resistance period, during which the capacity of the glands to respond to any new incoming stimuli is severely depressed.

This may provide a welcome period of rest and rehabilitation for the long overburdened physiological and metabolic processes, allowing them to regain the level of essential function from which they have deviated for so long under constant autonomic and endocrine stimulus. During this hiatus, the restoration of function can occur without disruption or interruption. Thus, the initiation of this artificial stress response may be the key by which fasting unlocks the body's own dormant healing energies.

Fasting and fertilization:

For conception to occur the female must be producing viable eggs during her monthly cycle and the male's sperm must be strong and healthy in order to fertilize the egg during intercourse. Infertility, which is quite simply the inability to conceive, is becoming more common and this "natural and simple" journey can be a difficult challenge given all the contributing factors to fertility. Factors such as diet, exercise, weight, health conditions, stress levels, emotional and mental states, genetics and a high toxic load in the blood stream all play a significant part in determining one's ability to conceive.

There are many ways to treat infertility however some treatments can be extremely off putting, stressful and expensive. One of the quickest and most effective ways at getting both the male and female ready for conception is by doing a fasting detox.

By undergoing a thorough cleanse the body has time to heal and regenerate itself on a cellular level. Fasting allows for all the toxins to be removed from the cells, hormones to be rebalanced, the liver to metabolize any excess hormones floating around the body such as xenoestrogens (found in chemicals, plastics and pesticides which create an imbalance in natural estrogen levels) and cortisol (stress hormone which can lead to inflammation, exhaustion, poor cellular function) which may be leading to infertility. Inflammation is decreased, all organs regenerated, blood sugars rebalanced, immune system boosted, nervous system rested and reproductive system balanced—amongst many other positive side effects—getting your body cleansed, detoxed, healthy and ready for fertility.

Fasting is also fantastic for couples that have undergone IVF without success or women who have been on various forms of synthetic contraception because it will "pull out" any excess or synthetic hormones, cleanse the liver, alkalize the blood stream and re boot the natural hormonal process of the body.

Fasting improves the fertility of men and women alike., Conducted by Dr. Samir Abbas and Dr. Abdullah Basalamah, Faculty of Medicine, King Abdul Aziz University, (1986) study on twenty-one people, eight of whom are healthy, and ten are suffering from a lack of sperms (oIigospermia), and three do not have sperms, and samples were taken from the blood, and semen, during the month of August, and September, and November, for semen analysis, and hormones following:

· Testosterone

· The prolactin

· LH L. H.

· Follicle-stimulating hormone (FSH)

In order to see the effect of the fasting month of Ramadan on a man's fertility, has shown results, that there are changes in the vitality of natural persons, which improves the performance of the male hormone (testosterone), but did not get the level of any rise dynamically during the three months of research, and that the volume of semen, and the total number of sperms, increased by a marked increase during the fasting month, noted the researchers of statistics university hospital, the number of pregnancies up to a significant rate in the month of September, also found that there is an improvement in the proportion of sperm live, and a decrease in the proportion of sperms dead during the month of fasting.

The follicle-stimulating hormone (FSH), is getting a marked increase during the month of Ramadan, compared to its level before and after fasting in the natural persons and at least the month of Shawwal in people who suffer from a lack of sperm, or lack thereof, and the hormone has to do with the manufacture vehicles steroidal in testicular tissue, It can also be attributed to the change in the level of testosterone to the change in the level of this hormone because the LH (LH) has increased markedly during fasting, and a lack of after the natural persons, as it did not register him any significant changes when sick people lack of sperms, and there is a shortage necessary when disease lack of sperm, this hormone has to do with the formation of sperms live in the testis, also recorded an increase in prolactin, during and after Ramadan when natural persons, and the lack of after fasting when patients lack of sperms, and high altitude when patients lack of sperms, compared with the other groups, this hormone has inhibitory effect on the output of testicular androgen.

The researchers concluded that the beneficial effect of fasting on the sperms, either by influencing the hormonal axis Hypothalamo - pituitary testicular, Or through a direct impact on the testicles.

Relationships between insulin and glucose metabolism and pituitary-ovarian functions in fasted heifers:

The effects of fasting between Days 8 and 16 of the estrous cycle on plasma concentrations of luteinizing hormone (LH), progesterone, cortisol, glucose and insulin were determined in 4 fasted and 4 control heifers during an estrous cycle of fasting and in the subsequent period after fasting. Cortisol levels were unaffected by fasting. Concentrations of insulin and glucose, however, were decreased (p less than 0.05) by 12 and 36 h, respectively, after fasting was begun and did not return to control values until 12 h (insulin) and 4 to 7 days (glucose) after fasting ended. Concentrations of progesterone were greater (p less than 0.05) in fasted than in control heifers from Day 10 to 15 of the estrous cycle during fasting, while LH levels were lower (p less than 0.01) in fasted than in control heifers during the last 24 h of fasting. Concentrations of LH increased (p less than 0.01) abruptly in fasted heifers in the first 4 h after they were refed on Day 16 of the fasted cycle. Concentrations (means +/- SEM) of LH also were greater (p less than 0.05) in fasted (11.2 +/- 2.6 ng/ml) than in control (4.7 +/- 1.2 ng/ml) heifers during estrus of the cycle after fasting; this elevated LH was preceded by a rebound response in insulin levels in the fasted-refed heifers, with insulin increasing from 176 +/- 35 pg/ml to 1302 +/- 280 pg/ml between refeeding and estrus of the cycle after fasting. Concentrations of LH, glucose and insulin were similar in both groups after Day 2 of the post fasting period. Concentrations of progesterone in two fasted heifers and controls were similar during the cycle after fasting, whereas concentrations in the other fasted heifers were less than 1 ng/ml until Day 10, indicating delayed ovulation and (or) reduced luteal function. Thus, aberrant pituitary and luteal functions in fasted heifers were associated with concurrent fasting-induced changes in insulin and glucose metabolism.

Fasting and thyroid hormones: conducted by Dr. Riad Soleimani (1988), a study on the impact of the fasting month of Ramadan on the work of the thyroid gland, and has been in the study was to determine the level of each of Thyroxin Plasma (Plasma Thyroxin: T4) and free thyroxin, and threonine tri-iodine (Triode - Thyroxin: T3) in stimulating hormone thyroid (TSH), when 28 healthy male, before Ramadan and beyond, has also been studying the effects of refraining from eating in the short term from dawn to sunset, There were no significant differences in tests of thyroid between these levels in the morning and evening, (after a period of fasting for 14 hours).

Did not show addition of any significant differences in the results of tests of the thyroid gland, which was conducted before and at the end of Ramadan, the researcher concluded that the fasting month of Ramadan by the men are in good health, did not change the standard ratios for the work of the thyroid gland.

In general, through the secretion of thyroxin hormones 3 and 4. The organization of the thyroid gland of the body all the pineal gland and anterior lobe of the pituitary gland, where carrying out when needed alert or activated.

In the case of an overactive thyroid gland, the patient feels Bohn in the muscles and nervous and irritable with a burning sensation and sweating and increased heartbeat.

It also records the weight loss and protruded in the eyes and swelling of the gland.

Treatment is antidot and surgery or radioactive iodine treatment. In the case of hypothyroidism or lack of activity the patient complains of a severe shortage in the level of activity of the body and lack of movement and gradual dullness and roughness of the skin, menstrual disorder in women. Be treated in this case compensation by giving the patient the hormone thyroxin.

For Ramadan, the doctors advise a patient with excessive thyroid activity fasting if his health is stable and if studiously to take medication in the case of lack of control over the disease has licensed physician often breakfast after examining the patient, especially in cases of disease.

For people with hypothyroidism, the patient deals with one pill of the hormone thyroxin and can just permission to fast and he took his medication at night.

For inflammatory thyroid distinguish between two types of infections: acute infections and usually allow because of the intensity to overcome the critical stage when the chronic inflammation may coexist with it can with the patient fasting.

Pituitary gland:

These relate thyroid gland with the hypothalamus through the pituitary together. There is a deficiency in the activity of the pituitary gland when it is not able to frontal lobe in manufacturing one or more of the hormone secreted by the hormones that are very essential and vital for the body, which have a very serious consequence for the physical growth and sexual maturation, and many of the vital functions. Symptoms include total symptoms consisting of thyroid disease and adrenal and nationality can arise this condition since birth as a result of oxygen deprivation, but it is often the result of a tumor pituitary or happens when you treat this tumor surgically or with radiation or inflammation of the pituitary gland and some injuries to the head and sometimes after severe bleeding during childbirth. Treatment lasts the length of life by administration the missing hormones.

For the disease, also called gigantism and acromegaly disease is a disease characterized by the gradual inflation of the hands, feet and bones of the head, the chest and the resulting increase in the secretion of growth hormone. Acromegaly produces disease in old age, unlike gigantism disease that develops before the age of puberty. The disease is caused by increased secretion of growth the hormone adenoma of the pituitary cells acidophilus. There are several lines of treatment: surgical treatment of radiation therapy and medical treatment.

For the Ramadan fast, these patients are usually advised not to fast.

Adrenal gland:

Located above the kidneys, and secret number of hormones such as cortisol and aldosterone and some reproductive hormones. Diseases of the adrenal gland are routine and non-common and come in the forefront Addison's disease and Cushing's disease and some tumors as melanoma.

Addison's disease: This disease occurs as a result of damage to the adrenal cortex, which leads to a lack of the hormone cortisol, which is known as inertial adrenal first. The symptoms of this disease: dizziness, joint pain, muscle weakness and fatigue and low blood pressure, digestive disorders with weight loss, as well as a change in skin color that tend to blackness in these patients.

For patients with Addison should not be fasting to avoid sharp declines in the rate of sugar in their blood.

Symptoms, short stature, high blood pressure, the emergence of obesity charges face that becomes rounded with the emergence of cheek redness and the occurrence of lines of purple on the hip, abdomen and thigh, with a feeling of general weakness, headache, and the instability of myself with a double collection semester, usually tends patients with Cushing's to diabetes. For this disease, the doctors do not advise infected with fasting.

Melanoma tumor: It is a rare disease, symptoms of swing numbers blood pressure, palpitations, sweating and weakness.

Advised not to fast when the melanoma tumor incidence, but the possibilities of treatment by surgery makes the patient recover his ability to perform this act of worship after his recovery.

Fasting is one of the safest and most appropriate methods for treating varicose veins. It does not destroy or coagulate the veins, which are accomplished by other means at the cost of overworking the deeper blood vessels, but it does heal varicose ulcers, helps to restore tonicity to the wall of the veins, reduce their size and provides freedom from pain in young people who are affected by varicosities of small to moderate size.

Full recovery is usually possible.

For the patient past middle age, with severe varicosities, definite improvement with comfort may be expected but complete recovery is rare in all cases, proper nutrition and adequate exercise after the fast are necessary to prevent excess fluid in tissues and assure continued improvement or maintenance of healthy tone of the walls of the veins.

When varicosities occur in the vein near the anus, as in hemorrhoids, fasting is also of much assistant.

During the fast there is little or no bowel action to occasion further irritation and healing of the affected areas is permitted. As early as 1854 Dr. Joel Shew stated that: "There is nothing in the world that will produce so greet relief in hemorrhoids as fasting."

In cases where to evacuate the bowels would put the patient into an agony, amounting almost to spasms there was marked improvement after only three or four days of fasting.

Dr. McCov described one case history of hemorrhoids in which the patient was unable to walk for several days before the fast because of severe pain that persisted day and night. Yet after only ten days of fasting, all signs of the hemorrhoids had disappeared, and the rectum seemed to be in quite a healthy condition. While writing on this same subject, Carrington stated: "I may add that I have observed some most striking examples of such cures myself."

Arthritis, rheumatism and gout as a rule respond quickly to the fast. Most patients experience freedom from severe arthritic pain within a few days after the fast is instituted.

There is gradual disappearance of the swelling and complete or partial absorption of the deformity by autolysis providing complete ossification of the joint is not present.

Dr. Casey A. Wood, Professor of Chemistry in the Medical Dept. of Bishop's College in Montreal, issued a report concerning seven case histories of acute articular rheumatism.

These patients were speedily restored to health during four to eight days of fasting. Dr. Wood also mentioned forty other similar cases from his own private practice in which recovery from this disease was achieved, and in no instance was it necessary to fast longer than ten days.

However, patients affected by severe chronic arthritis of long standing must often undertake longer fasts. Those who are so crippled that they are unable to walk alone, comb their hair or even feed themselves often achieve restoration of considerable motion to the stiffened joints during a single fast, although complete recovery (when this is possible) in some of these cases may require a second fast.

Of the one hundred and more pathological conditions which affect the skin, most can be treated successfully with fasting.

Even in so serious a condition as leprosy, the skin ulcerations nodules have disappeared in just a few weeks of fasting and sunbathing.

For simple acne and other common skin diseases, recovery tends to be more rapid, with most cases responding to care in one to two weeks or less. Eczema and severe skin diseases, however, may require longer fasts. In all cases, improvement is limited to the removal of swelling, inflammation, excess scaly tissue, ulcerations, etc.

For this reason early treatment in many cases is recommended.

Once severe scar tissue has formed, little or nothing can be done to restore the original skin texture.

CHAPTER 10

The effect of fasting on eye diseases

Prognosis in the case of many eye diseases is good if fasting is employed. Numerous cases of visual defects have been completely remedied by fasting, though some mechanical defects cannot be corrected of course, and certain eye ailments require aid which fasting cannot give.

When the muscles of the eyes suffer from a lack of tone, strength, flexibility, suppleness and coordination, special eye exercises will give more benefit than fasting, though fasting may be used to supplement this treatment.

Among the eye conditions for which fasting is often a particular remedy are cataract, congestion of the conjunctiva, catarrhal and granular conjunctivitis, glaucoma, iritis, keratitis and stye. Early cataract generally disappears on the fast; advanced cases may disappear, but recovery is much less certain.

Dr. Shelton records one case in which blindness of one eye (due to cataract) completely disappeared on a fast of 18 days. Dr. Gerald Benesh reports equal success in treating a complete cataract, which yielded to a 21 day fast.

The forms of conjunctivitis require only cleanliness and fasting for recovery, with short fasts in acute cases and long fasts in chronic cases.

When glaucoma exists, the hardness of the eye tends to disappear, with the excessive fluid being absorbed, on fasts of two or three weeks in duration.

In advanced cases, when complete atrophy is present, the prognosis is not favorable, with blindness the usual result.

Iritis, keratitis and stye need only fasting, cleanliness and rest, with recovery the general rule unless previous suppressive treatment leaves permanent damage to sight.

Respiratory ailments respond quickly to the fast. Hay fever improves in virtually all cases without any change of climate.

Patients with catarrh recover on the fast, although eliminations may increase temporarily on the early days of the fast.

Polyps, which may be present, are absorbed; the thickened membranes return to their normal thickness, though the atrophied structures of advanced catarrh cannot he rebuilt.

CHAPTER 11

The effect of fasting on respiratory diseases

Sinusitis responds readily to the fast; only a few days of fasting will bring relief in some cases; in others, long fasts may be necessary.

Chronic laryngitis yields quickly to the fast. Chronic cases of asthma usually attain much relief within just a few days of fasting, with complete recovery in a matter of weeks.

Those asthmatics that are unable to sleep lying in bed and consequently sleep in a sitting position are usually relieved sufficiently within 36 hours without food to sleep in bed. Dr. Benesh refers to different patients recovering from severe and longstanding asthma on fasts of different duration.

One case required two fasts of longstanding asthma on fasts of different duration. And 7 days; the third fasted 26 days, and two fasts of 23 and 26 days were necessary in the most advanced case.

Of the hundreds of asthmatics treated by Dr. Shelton with fasting, only three failed to recover.

Congestion of the lungs is rapidly and safely remedied in all cases through fasting, and bronchitis responds equally well to treatment.

The most important respiratory disease, tuberculosis of the lungs, has often been treated with the fast. In the vast majority of cases the prognosis is very favorable. While fasting, the tubercular cough usually becomes very mild or altogether disappears.

In some cases much improvement occurs on the fast, followed by complete recovery during a period of proper nutrition with adequate fresh air and careful exposure to sunlight.

A short fasting period is usually given preference in tuberculosis cases because of the difficulty some patients have had in gaining weight after long fasts.

Yet, a number of patients have recovered during long fasts and have returned to normal weight.

It is possible that the difficulties which occurred in other cases were due to poor control of the dietary habits after fasting.

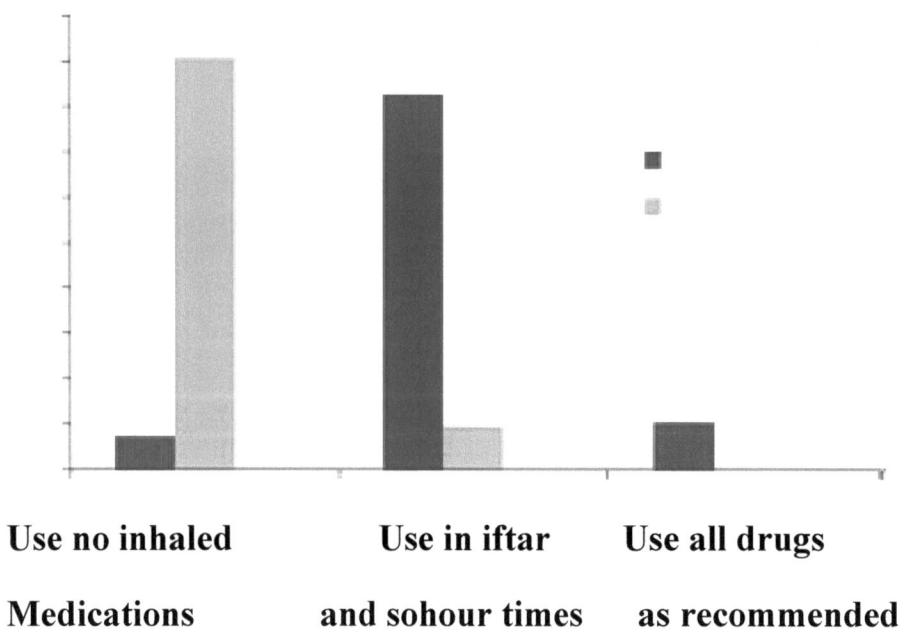

Use no inhaled   **Use in iftar**   **Use all drugs**

Medications   **and sohour times**   **as recommended**

Use of inhaled medications during Ramadan of patients with asthma and COPD.

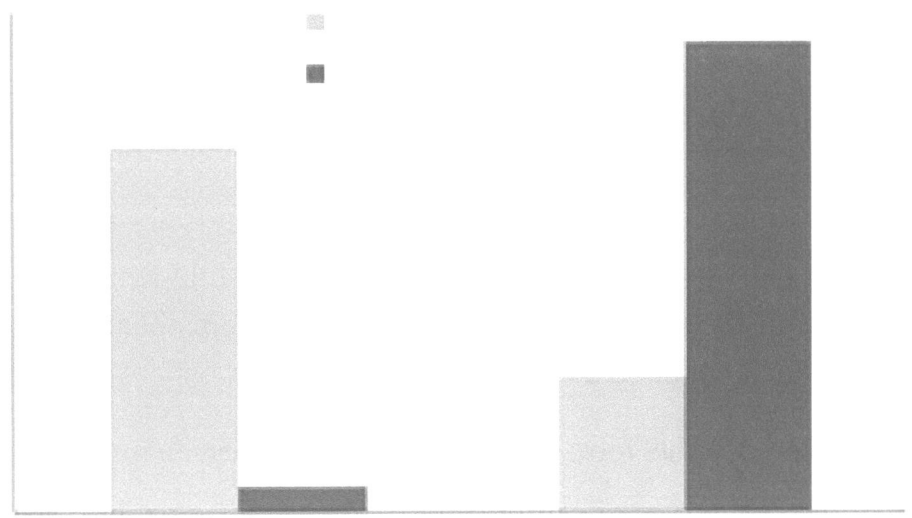

Use reliever as needed any time
needed

No use of reliever even as

COPD ● **Asthma**

CHAPTER 12

Fasting and infectious diseases

Typhoid fever patients recover in about two weeks while fasting in absence of most of the distressing symptoms which result from feeding and giving medication to such patients.

Smallpox takes only the form of a light disease when fasting is instituted immediately.

There is only very slight itching, no complications, and very rarely any pitting at all.

In cases of scarlet fever, the rash disappears within four to seven days and the fever is gone by the fourth day.

Mumps disappear within six to ten days of fasting, with no danger of complications.

Regarding rheumatic fever, Dr. Weger claims that "in no case in which food was withheld from the onset did the temperature remain above normal for longer than ten days, and recovery was prompt without merging into the sub-acute and chronic stage."

In the case of influenza, Dr. Weger points to the "rapid decline of all symptoms and abatement of temperature usually within three days," while fasting, with no mortality rate at all.

Erysipelas, he declares, is "readily checked without pursuing its usual round-trip course." Fever disappears on the third or fourth day, with no abscesses or secondary infections. Dr. Weger not only refers to recovery from malaria "in all stages" but states that no relapses "have been reported on return from fever-infested surroundings."

There are no age barriers to fasting. Both aged individuals and young children have fasted with great benefit.

Even infants may be placed on short fasts, and there is one record of a 2-year-old child fasting to recovery from poliomyelitis, with paralysis, on a 47-day fast, during which time the weight fell from 32 pounds to 15 pounds. Obviously such long fasts in children are the exception rather than the general rule, and they are not always to be recommended.

Nor is long fasting often necessary during childhood, most children's diseases disappearing rapidly during short fasts.

Fasting is of supreme importance in the treatment of all cases of poliomyelitis.

In the acute form the prognosis as regards life is good, with a much lower death rate than follows either the Kenny treatment or orthodox treatment.

Cases of permanent disability are almost unknown when fasting is employed, with all paralysis rapidly disappearing within a weeks in most cases.

In an average of 98 percent of all recovery is complete while fasting or shortly after the fast.

When chronic anterior poliomyelitis is present the prognosis is less favorable, though further degeneration is usually checked and the life is prolonged.

Bulbar paralysis, a less common form of poliomyelitis, may end fatally no matter what form of treatment is given. Fasting, however, still gives the best chance of recovery and prolongation of life.

CHAPTER 13

Fasting and patients with urinary tract problems

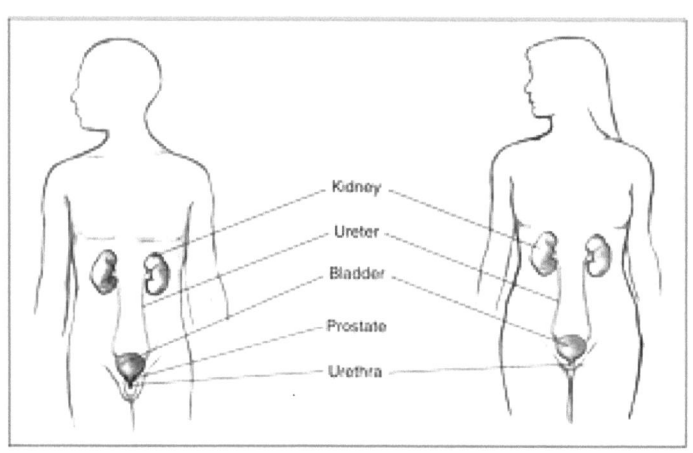

Male and female urinary tracts.

The doctors still believe that fasting affects urinary tract disease, especially for those who are suffering from gallstones, or kidney failure. Patients are advised to eat mushrooms and drink large amounts of fluids.

It has been proven otherwise, it might have been fasting reason not to be some of the stones, and melt some salts did not affect fasting never even on those who suffer from the most serious diseases of the urinary system, renal failure, a disease with repeated washing.

Conducted by Dr. Fahim Abdul Rahim and his colleagues at the Faculty of Medicine of Al-Azhar (1986), in search of the effect of the fasting month of Ramadan on the work and functions of the kidneys when ordinary people, and in patients with certain diseases of the urinary system, or disease to be gravel kidney (Renal calculi), and the study included ten patients urology, and fifteen patients with gravel, in addition to ten ordinary people for comparison, has been through all of the periods of fasting & B sampling of urine, and analyzed to determine the proportion of calcium, sodium, potassium, urea, creatinine, and uric acid.

The result of the effect of fasting on these elements is as follows:

Important event shortage in urine volume, and an increase in the density of quality, with all the groups surveyed, and very minor changes have occurred in the components of serum calcium, sodium, potassium, uric acid, creatinine, and urea.

There has been a slight increase in calcium in the urine.

Accordingly, it has been the change in the components of the vaccine among all groups surveyed slight, insignificant, however, that the changes in the components of urine during fasting, may prevent the formation of stones, due to lack of calcium in the urine, and increased sodium and potassium, which was attributed greater in those who suffer from the gravel, and in patients with urinary tract disease.

The researchers concluded from this that fasting did not adversely affect the patient groups that included this study, and those who suffer from either the formation of stones in college as well as the potential impact of fasting to prevent the stones formation. The increase in specific gravity of urine due to increased secretion of urea, which is 80% of the solutes in the urine, and urea glue spread on helping non-deposition of urine salts that are urinary tract stones.

A study on patients with chronic dialysis fasted during Ramadan and proved that there was no significant change in the proportion of urea, creatinine, sodium, bicarbonate, and calcium and phosphorus, but found a significant increase on the proportion of potassium in the blood; the researchers attributed this to the potassium-rich drinks after breakfast.

Fasting has been used with success in the treatment of various forms of sexual disorders and venereal diseases.

Dr. Hazzard points out that the bacillus of gonorrhea "cannot long exist if the products of elimination are normal, and if cleanliness, especially of the female, is correctly observed." She states that the "irritating symptoms of local venereal infection yield to treatment (fasting) in a few days, and convalescence brings no supervening annoyance as expressed in urethral stricture, prostatic congestion, etc."

Regarding syphilis, Dr. Shew wrote that "The hunger-cure is nowhere more applicable."

The high medical authority, Dr. Robert Bartholow, also pointed out the value of fasting in such cases. Dr. Shelton states that "without exception" his patients with syphilis "have gotten well in four to eight weeks under hygienic care."

Dr. Tilden refers to recovery from syphilis "in from six weeks to two months without aftermaths of any kind" when the fasting treatment, followed by correct diet, is employed.

Dr. Weger claims that the "local lesions of the first-stage heal with startling rapidity' and that "pharyngeal, labial, and buccal ulcerations frequently disappear before the tenth day of fasting."

In treating diseases of the female reproductive system, fasting relieves congestion, removes infection, relaxes tissues and restores tone to the affected area.

Abnormal growths of the womb tend to be partially or completely absorbed during the fast.

The supposed need for surgical operation, with its attendant dangers and disadvantages, is thus reduced or eliminated when diseases of the female organs occur. In such simple conditions as painful and excessive menstruation, fasting is also of distinct value. Dr. Hazzard stated that "from one to three day's abstinence from food will correct excessive menstruation, and, when no mechanical defect is present relief is obtained within twenty-four hours when the flow is accompanied by pain."

Diabetes was first treated with fasting by the famous French clinician, A. Guelpa, of Paris. Dr. Guelpa noted that fasting for three or four successive days rendered the urine of patient with severe diabetes sugar-free, and effected pronounced improvement in the state of health, with no aggravation of the disease in any case.

The American physician Dr. Heinrich Stern was next to treat diabetes with fasting and reduced nutritional intake, and his many hundreds of patients as a rule responded favorably. Dr. Stern found though there were individual cases of the severest types of diabetes "which no amount of fasting would render sugar-free." The majority of patients "cease to excrete sugar within forty-eight to sixty hours;' with an occasional patient fasting six days or longer before the glycosuria symptom disappeared. In approximately seventy-five percent of all cases the urine also rendered free from ketones, though this required a longer period of fasting. Dr. Frederick Allen of the Rockefeller Institute has also employed the "starvation treatment" of diabetes, and his outstanding work with fasting and restricted diet in 1915 effected a 60 percent reduction in deaths from diabetic coma.

In healthy persons, fasting Ramadan does not induce abnormalities of urinary volume, osmolality, pH, and solute and electrolyte excretion. Changes in serum urea and creatinine are usually insignificant, and the alterations in serum sodium and potassium are negligible. However, in chronic kidney disease (CKD) patients, Ramadan fasting is shown to induce adverse impact on renal function.

Previous studies have reported that carbohydrate metabolism is slowed down by Ramadan fasting in human subjects while fat oxidation is significantly increased. On the other hand, there are observations suggesting that similar types of Ramadan type fasting in the rat models result in intense provocation of enzymes engaged in several metabolic activities such as the tricarboxylic acid cycle, gluconeogenesis, and glycolysis in the gastrointestinal tract as well as in the liver. Moreover, in rat models, 30 day-Ramadan-type fasting resulted in a decrease of blood cholesterol and glucose as well as a minor lowering of body weight as observed after Ramadan fasting in human subjects. Whole blood lactate and pyruvate levels also fell during Ramadan fasting in human subjects. Although a variety of changes in urine volume, osmolarity, solutes, ions, and urea were observed after Ramadan fasting in humans, there is no evidence of any adverse impact on kidney functions.

While it is presumed that prolonged intermittent abstinence from water and food concomitantly for 12 hours daily for 30 days may stress the kidneys and alter their metabolic and transport functions, serum creatinine and blood urea nitrogen as well as creatinine clearance were not unaltered by this feeding pattern, suggesting that normal kidney function remains intact.

Prolonged intermittent Ramadan type fasting induces a significant decrease in lactate dehydrogenase and malate dehydrogenase activities in renal cortex and medulla, as well as the enzymes involved in both the glucose degradation and production including glucose-6-phosphatase and fructose-1, 6-bisphosphatas. In addition, reversible increased liver and intestine enzymatic activities have also been reported during Ramadan type fasting.

Table 1 - First morning urine albumin concentration, volume, fasting blood glucose and
HbA_1 of 50 IDDM patients.

Data for urinary albumin and first morning urine volume are reported as median (range)
(Friedman test). The other data are reported as means ± SD. There were no statistical
differences between samples for any of the variables studied (Student t-test).

Variables	Samples		
	First	Second	Third
Urinary albumin (µg/ml)	6.1 (1-95)	5.8 (1.1-80)	6.2 (1.2-75)
Urine volume (ml)	222.5 (27-910)	210 (5-1120)	200 (25-640)
Glucose (mg/dl)	181.9 ± 93.6		194.6 ± 104.7
HbA_1 (%)	8.4 ± 1.3		8.8 ± 1.5

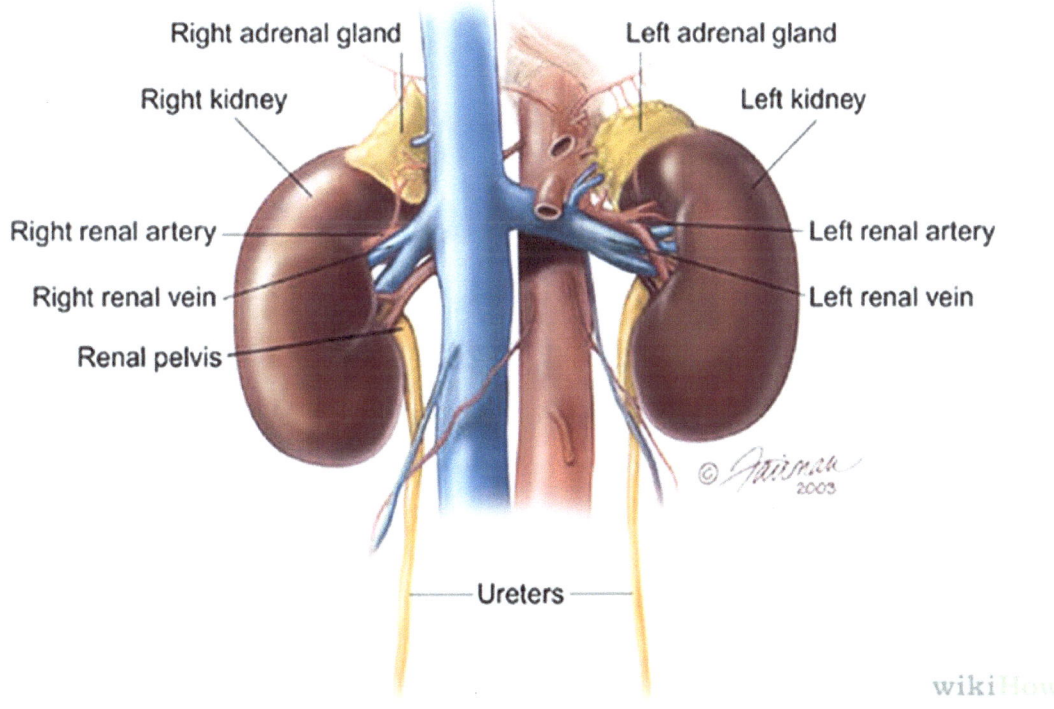

Understand a Kidney-Cleansing Fast Step.

CHAPTER 14

Fasting and transplantation

Transplant patients are at increased risk of adverse effects related to fasting due to their underlying illness and immunosuppressive medication. Prior to the commencement of Ramadan Muslim patients ask their doctors whether they can fast. The major concern in these patients is that if dehydration and accumulation of metabolites may result in irreversible deterioration in renal function or facilitate rejection episodes via inducing changes in immune system. One study did not find any change in circulating immune complexes during Ramadan fasting in the normal population, and another reported a decrease in complement C3 levels and an increase in C4 levels in renal transplant recipients.

With increasing the number of renal transplants performed in Islamic countries as well as improved quality of life, the question of the safety of fasting Ramadan is asked more often. Several investigations have addressed this issue and found no significant adverse effects of Ramadan fasting on transplant patients or allografts; Argani studied 24 patients and found no significant increase in body weight, blood pressure, 24-hour urine volume, protein to urine creatinine ratio or blood urea nitrogen. In addition, T-cell and white cell counts, hemoglobin levels, and low density lipoprotein did not change significantly after completion of 30 days of Ramadan fasting. B cells counts, serum IgM concentration, serum C 3 levels, and serum very-low-density lipoproteins value all significantly decreased after fasting compared to pre-fast period. Higher levels of high density lipoprotein and serum C4 values were also observed after Ramadan fasting. The authors finally concluded that Ramadan fasting was not harmful to stable renal transplant patients with a 12-hour fasting pattern. However, they proposed that patients should be observed carefully by their physicians while fasting.

Einollahi studied 19 kidney transplant recipients who voluntarily fasted Ramadan and compared them with 20 matched recipients who did not fast. All the patients had serum creatinine values below 1.5 mg/dL at entry to the study. No significant change in serum creatinine concentrations before and after Ramadan was observed in both groups. The authors concluded safety of fasting Ramadan in recipients with stable renal function and followed it with another study of 41 Ramadan fasting kidney transplant recipients who were compared to matched controls. The mean of estimated glomerular filtration rate (GFR) did not significantly change after 30 days of fasting (72.8 ± 27.8 and 73.1 ± 29.3 mL/min in the fasting group, and 73.4 ± 18.8 and 73.1 ± 18.5 mL/min in the controls, pre and post 30 days of fasting, respectively). The authors concluded that for patients with GFR higher than 60 mL/min, Ramadan fasting did not cause impairment of allograft function.

Abdualla studied 17 renal transplant recipients with normal function and 6 with stable but impaired allograft function (plasma creatinine levels not exceeding 300 mmol/L). No significant changes were observed in any of the studied parameters before, during, and after Ramadan. The authors concluded that fasting Ramadan did not cause any significant adverse effects on kidney transplant recipients with normal or impaired graft function and suggested that it is safe for those patients to fast during Ramadan after one year of renal transplantation.

Ghalib studied 68 renal transplant recipients; 35 patients in a fasting study group and 33 in a non-fasting control group. When the fasters acted as their own controls, the mean GFR after the third Ramadan did not differ significantly from that at baseline (56.4 and 55.4 mL/min). The differences in GFR over this period remained insignificant after multivariate adjustment for age, presence of diabetes mellitus (DM), baseline GFR, proteinuria, or duration postransplant. Furthermore, no rejection episodes or renal function deterioration were observed during or soon after Ramadan.

Said studied 145 kidney transplant recipients (age 18 to 64 years); 71 patients fasted during Ramadan while 74 did not. The serum creatinine and blood urea did not show any significant change between the two groups before and after fasting. There was a tendency for higher blood sugar in patients with types I diabetes mellitus. Cyclosporine toxicity was observed in two fasters, and acute rejection episodes occurred in other two, urinary tract infection occurred in two more. No graft or patient loss occurred in any of the groups. Authors finally concluded that fasting Ramadan by kidney transplant recipients with normal kidney function is safe, but diabetic patients should exercise more caution during fasting.

Finally Boobes studied 22 (12 women) kidney transplant patients with stable kidney functions and voluntarily chose to fast Ramadan. Body weight, blood pressure, kidney function tests, blood sugar, lipid profile, and cyclosporine levels remained stable after Ramadan fasting, and the authors concluded that it is safe for kidney transplant recipients of more than one year and stable graft function to fast Ramadan. However, they cautioned about possible adverse impact of fasting on the patients with moderate to severe impaired renal function despite nonspecific findings.

Based on this literature review, the general belief among medical professionals in transplantation is to allow fasting when the transplanted kidney graft is functioning well for at least one year. The overall number of transplant patients fasting during Ramadan studied in all the reviewed articles was 213 patients, which may not be large enough to have a final conclusion. However, none of the studies found any significant adverse effects related to Ramadan type fasting. Although two studies, suggested preserving Ramadan fasting to patients without impaired allograft function, no evidence was presented in any of them.

Defining specific allograft function values as safe levels for Ramadan fasting is also of extreme relevance, since none of the studies defined renal function level for safe fasting; GFR level ≥ 60 mL/min was not based on scientific findings, but a mere prediction.

All the existing literature was on kidney transplant recipients and we did not find any study in other transplant patients. This may be due to the better quality of life and larger patient population in kidney transplant group than other organ recipients.

One of the major limitations of the current studies is that they do not mention the compliance of the patients for all the 30 days of fasting and this may impose an obstacle in discussing the results.

We conclude that Ramadan fasting represents no major adverse effect on kidney allografts in kidney transplant recipients. However, larger studies targeting distinct groups of patients (for example diabetic patients) and describing more precisely the fasting process of patients are required to better evaluate the impact of Ramadan fasting on this population.

Simple gall bladder and bile duct infection is completely remedied during fasts of short to moderate duration. The pus is removed, the inflammation subsides and the tissues are healed during this physiological rest. When stones have formed in the gall bladder, somewhat longer fasts may be required but recovery is to be expected.

The patient with gallstones finds relief from severe pain after the first few days of the fast, although complete recovery in the more advanced cases may require up to 20 to 25 days of abstinence from food. During the fast, the stones soften, later disintegrate and then pass through the bile duct into the small intestine.

Some pain may occur during the passage of stones but this does not involve the extreme discomfort frequently experienced prior to the fast.

CHAPTER 15

Fasting during pregnancy and lactation

The only periods of life in which the use of fasting may be questioned are those of lactation and pregnancy. Fasting stops the secretion of milk and hence prevents the mother from nursing her child. During pregnancy long fasts to remedy chronic diseases are certainly inadvisable, though when acute disease exists, there may be a short fast until most or all of the symptoms subside.

Clearly, in terms of strict efficiency, fasting is of exceptional value as a therapeutic measure. It is in no sense a cure-all, nor is it the only method whereby health can be restored. As was noted, some conditions in their advanced stages do not always recover on the fast. Further, the same results which often occur while fasting may occur by employing certain diets, though the latter method frequently is much less precise and incomparably slower than the fast. For speed and certainty in recovery the fast has no equal in the cases of most diseases, as the employment of fasting in thousands of cases clearly shown. As regards efficiency, it is in a class by itself.

In another volume we have called attention to the fact that chronic "disease," even that form called tuberculosis, frequently abates during pregnancy. Significant changes, developmental changes akin to those of puberty and adolescence, take place in a woman's body during pregnancy. Weak hearts, weak lungs, weak kidneys, weak nervous systems are strengthened. Glands long dormant awaken to activity. Her whole body undergoes a strengthening, renovating process.

This is the meaning of the nausea, vomiting, ("morning sickness"), lack of appetite and other symptoms that so many women experience during the early weeks of pregnancy. No woman in good health, who is living sensibly, ever has the slightest trace of these symptoms. No woman who has undergone a thorough renovation just prior to becoming pregnant, and who lives sensibly during this time, ever experiences these "symptoms of pregnancy."

They are not signs of pregnancy. They are signs of renovation. They indicate that nature is undertaking a house cleaning, that the body is to be put into its best shape preparatory to pregnancy and parturition. If they are heeded all will be well. If they are not heeded, life will usually succeed in her work in spite of opposition and interference. Sometimes she fails. Always her success is more complete and more satisfactory if we cooperate with her.

The development of these symptoms is a sure sign that a house-cleaning is necessary. When anorexia, nausea and vomiting develop, absolutely no food but water should be taken until these have disappeared and there is a distinct call for food. There should be no fears about fasting. You may be sure that these symptoms will end and nature will call for food as soon as her renovating work is completed and long before there has been any damage to mother or fetus. A fast is just what she is calling for in the plainest possible manner, and a fast she usually gets even if she has to keep throwing the food back into the woman's face as often as she eats it for days. Rest is called for as loudly as the fast and should be had.

If this renovating work is permitted full sway and the woman will eat and live sensibly, afterward, there will be no necessity for another fast during pregnancy. She will continue in good health. But if she "eats for two" (six), and lives the conventional, unhygienic life, she will suffer from a sour stomach, gas, dizziness, headaches, constipation and frequently more serious difficulties. She may develop an acute "disease." In such a case the hygiene of the "disease" is the same as it would be were it to develop in any other period of life. The pregnant woman should not hesitate to fast for as long as nature indicates if she is suffering with an acute eliminating crisis. Let her be assured that to do so will shorten her period of illness, and that it will harm neither her nor her child. On the other hand, to eat will not help either her or the child.

The ridiculous advice to pregnant mothers to "eat for two," is beginning to lose its assumed validity. Suppose a baby weighs nine pounds at birth (three pounds too much); this is an average gain of a pound a month during the period of pregnancy. To meet the requirements of the baby growing at such a relatively slow rate, the mother is urged to eat two, three or more extra pounds of food a day. Instead of this being helpful to her and the evolving child, it helps to make her sick, provides for a fat, hence oversized baby, reduces the health and elasticity of her tissues, and provides for great pains in childbirth. During pregnancy she has nausea, vomiting, sour stomach, swollen ankles, varicose veins, hemorrhoids, eclampsia, etc., as a consequence of such unintelligent eating.

In vomiting during pregnancy, physicians are afraid of both starvation and dehydration, hence they keep the woman plied with fluids and foods. All manners of clean and unclean things are introduced into the woman's stomach, in addition to the inordinate drugging that usually accompanies such cases when cared for by regular physicians. There should be no wonder that the vomiting continues.

There is no danger of starvation and we may be sure that the vomiting will cease before any marked or dangerous dehydration can occur, providing the woman is not fed. Indeed, in the absence of food, she will usually be able to take water. Nothing succeeds like fasting in morning sickness.

Chronic "disease" should not be handled differently during pregnancy to the manner in which it is handled at other times. The author would object to a long fast in chronic "disease" during this period. There can, however, be no objection to a short fast, but a long fast involves elements that one should seek to avoid.

Dr. Hazzard says: "When pregnant woman fasts, her tissues, even including such essential ones as the heart and brain, will be utilized as may be necessary to properly nourish the child." This can be true only after the exhaustion of her internal reserves; for, true to the principle that the tissues are sacrificed in inverse order to their importance, the essential organs are not damaged until it becomes necessary to sacrifice them for the child. But a woman does not want to lose her hair, or nails, or teeth, nor should she be asked to where this can be avoided. Under the modern plan of feeding, most women lose a tooth and develop a few cavities during pregnancy, anyway.

A short fast, where one is necessary, or will be of benefit, should be entered upon without hesitancy by the pregnant woman suffering with a chronic "disease," but a long one should be avoided unless acute "disease "makes it necessary. Feeding in acute "disease" does not feed, anyway.

Many published and online sources confirm that Muslim women are exempt from fasting Ramadan during pregnancy (Josooph, 2004; Malik, Mubarak, & Hussein, 1996; Pearce & Mayho, 2004; Sulimani, 1991). This exemption is likely based on the interpretation that fasting during pregnancy causes hardship and difficulties the same way illness does. The Qur'an states "[fasting for] a limited number of days. So whoever among you is ill, or on a journey [during them]-then an equal number of other days [are to be made up]. And upon those who are able [to fast but with hardship]-a ransom [as substitute] of feeding a poor person [each day]" (The Qur'an, 2007; S 2, V 183).

An explicit exemption for pregnant women was found in the Hadith Sharif referred to by Abdullah Ibn Abbas "If a pregnant women fears for herself (i.e., for her health) or the breastfeeding woman fears for her child in Ramadan, they should break their fast and feed a poor person for each day (they miss) and they do not have to make up the fast" (Hallaq, 2007, p. 550). Hadith Sharif is a report of saying based on the teachings and practices of the prophet Muhammad. It is considered to be a main source of religious law after Qur'an.

Islam protects the child even before its birth which explains why Muslim scholars exempt a pregnant woman if she believes that fasting may cause harm to her health and/or to her unborn baby (Josooph 2004). Some scholars emphasize the need to make up the missed days once the pregnancy is over while others emphasize giving money and food to the poor or needy or the ransom.

A limited number of studies have investigated the unclear effect of fasting on the health status of the mother and her unborn baby during pregnancy.

Some research findings demonstrated adverse effects of fasting on the mother and her unborn baby. For example in a study by Rabinerson, Dicker, Kaplan, Ben-Rafael, and Dekel (2000), an increased risk of hyperemesis gravid arum in fasting women during the first month of pregnancy was found. In another study by Malhotra, Scott, Scott, Gee, and Wharton (1989), the maternal cortisol of fasting women was elevated. Mirghani, Weerasinghe, Ezimokhani, and Smith (2003) found a reduction in fetal breathing movements due to the low level of blood glucose concentration in fasting pregnant mothers. In a more recent study, Mirghani, Weerasinghe, Smith, and Ezimokhani (2004) found a reduction in fetal biophysical profile in fasting pregnant mothers, which could indicate a certain level of fetal compromise. Finally, Bandyopadhyay, Thakur, Ray, and Kumar (2005) stated that insufficient fluid intake during pregnancy due to fasting increases Muslim women's prevalence of urinary tract infections.

Other studies demonstrated that fasting has no effect on the unborn baby. For example, Cross, Eminson, and Wharton (1990) found that maternal fasting during Ramadan did not affect the birth weight of babies born at full term. In another study by Kavehmanesh and Abolghasemi (2004) maternal fasting, during Ramadan, did not affect neonatal birth weight. Finally, Dikensoy (2008) found that maternal fasting did not lead to ketonemia or ketonuria in pregnant women. They also found that it did not affect intrauterine fetal development or the fetus's health.

Regardless of the effect of fasting on the health status of the mothers and their unborn babies, some pregnant Muslim women may choose to fast. For example, in a study by Josooph (2004) most Muslim women chose to fast during pregnancy with support from their spouses and other family members. However, these women lacked the basic religious knowledge regarding Islamic law of fasting during pregnancy. In another study by Robinson and Raisler (2005), pregnant Muslim women avoided discussing fasting with their healthcare providers for fear of being treated disrespectfully or advised against fasting.

If fasting is necessary during lactation, it should be done, but if not essential it should be avoided, for the reason that it stops the secretion of milk and even the diminution of this secretion resulting from a fast of three or four days is seldom overcome by a return to eating.

If only one of the essential elements of nutrition is withdrawn from the diet of hens, they immediately cease lying. By these means the great amount of food lost to the body through the production of eggs is conserved and life prolonged. A similar thing is seen in fasting mammals in which milk production ceases. In all animals, scarcity of food limits reproduction.

Many published and online sources exempt Muslim women from fasting while breastfeeding. They base their exemption on the fact that Islam values life and seeks to fulfill and satisfy the child's vital needs; therefore, a woman is permitted to break a fast to save a life. If fasting is going to harm the infant then the Muslim mother should break her fast to save the life of her infant who depends on her breast milk for nourishment.

Despite this clear exemption, some Muslim women may elect to fast Ramadan while breastfeeding. For example, in a study by Ertem (2001) the attitudes and practices of breastfeeding mothers regarding fasting during Ramadan were investigated. They found that 22% of breastfeeding mothers perceived a decrease in their breast milk production, and 23% reported increasing the amount of infant supplements during fasting. Most mothers (76%) believed that fasting decreased their breast milk and 65% believed that breastfeeding mothers should not fast. However, 41% of the mothers who believed that fasting decrease breast milk production and 34% of those who believed that breastfeeding mothers should not fast, were fasting. Many Muslim women choose to fast during Ramadan do it for spiritual reasons or because they find it more difficult to fast alone at a later time if they have to make up the missed days (Cross-Sudworth, 2007).

There is a lack of knowledge about the actual effects of fasting while breastfeeding on the mother-infant relationship and consequently the infant's health. Research states that fasting causes physiological changes such as "sleepiness, lack of concentration, weakness, exaggerated responsiveness, irritability, nervousness and aggressiveness" (Afifi, 1997, p. 232). The effect of such changes on the breastfeeding mother and her production of breast milk needs to be investigated.

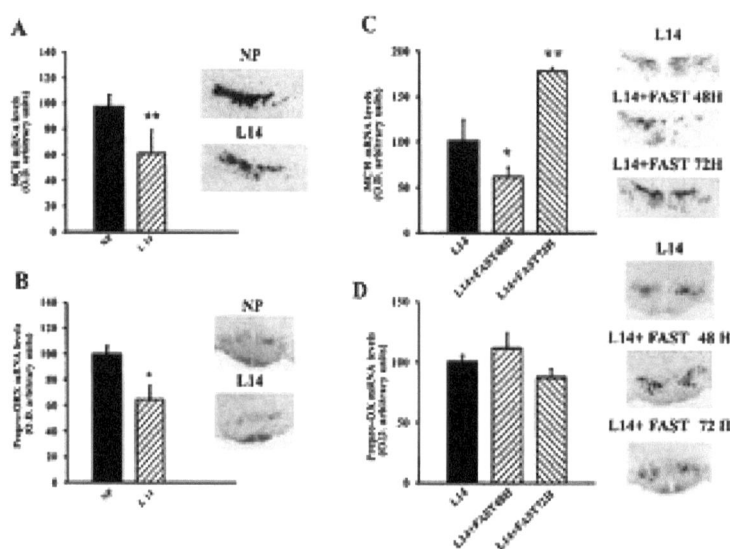

A) MCH and B) prepro-OX mRNA levels in the LH of nonpregnant (NP) and lactating (L14) rats. Data (mean±SE) were expressed as % change in relation to nonpregnant rats. P<0.05 and P<0.01 vs. nonpregnant animals. C) MCH and D) prepro-OX mRNA levels in fed (L14) and 48 and 72 h fasted lactating rats (L14+FAST 48H and L14+FAST72H). Data (mean±SE) were expressed as % change in relation to lactating rats fed ad libitum. P<0.05 and P <0.01 vs. fed animals. A—D) Right panels: Auto radiographic images of representative coronal brain sections incubated with a ^{35}S -labeled antisense oligonucleotide for MCH, or a ^{35}S -labeled antisense prepro-OX mRNA probe at the level of the LH.

CHAPTER 16

Fasting and body temperature

When we observe body temperature during a fast, we are presented with a paradoxical series of phenomena which prove both interesting and highly instructive. For example, temperature tends to remain normal in most cases of fasters suffering with chronic disease, to fall in acute disease and to rise in those patients who have sub-normal temperature. Benedict points out that during the fast, for a period of seven days at least, there is an occasional tendency for it to increase as the fast progresses.

Temperature does not rise as high in fever patients who are not fed as it does in the same patients when fed. Invariably, the temperature falls to normal as the fast progresses. Indeed, in acute "disease," where there is high temperature, the fever subsides somewhat as soon as eating is discontinued and seldom rises high thereafter.

In rare cases of chronic disease there is sub-normal temperature. This is most likely to be observed in the morning before the patient has become active. It is striking evidence of the value of the fast that in these patients, as the fast nears its natural termination, the temperature rises to normal and remains there. In those chronic sufferers whose temperature is habitually below normal, it will surely but slowly rise until it reaches normal by the time the fast naturally ends. "Thus," says Carrington, "supposing the patient's temperature to be 93.8° at the commencement of the fast, it will gradually rise until about 98.4° is reached—though the fast may have extended over forty or more days…. Time after time, in case after case, I have watched this gradual rise in the bodily temperature of the patient, and in every case the temperature has not failed to rise as the fast progressed. At first, it is true, the temperature sometimes tends to fall, but let the fast be persisted in, and a return or rise to normal will occur in every case."

Carrington records several cases where temperature was subnormal while eating, but gradually returned to normal while fasting. In some of these, premature eating resulted in an immediate drop in temperature. One case he records had a temperature below 94° F. before the fast. At the end of a thirty-four days fast the temperature had nearly reached the normal standard.

A. Rabagliatti, M.A., M.D., F.R.C.S., Edinburgh, made this same discovery, and says of it, "In point of fact, I raised the temperature of a man who was, besides thin, emaciated, and attenuated by constant vomiting, lasting for seven years, from 96° F. to 98.4° F. by advising him to fast for thirty-five days. On the 28th day his temperature had risen to normal, and remained so." —*Air, Food and Exercise*, p. 261.

Low temperature is often the result of too much food, or lowered vitality due to habitual over-eating. The case just quoted from Dr. Rabagliatti was, as he remarks, "dying on the plan of frequent feeding." He lost 13 pounds during the fast and gained health although he had been sick and taking a "highly nourishing diet" for seven years. Carrington noted a few instances of long fasts where the temperature dropped a degree or two immediately upon resuming eating.

Dr. Hazzard records a case in which body temperature was constantly at ninety-four degrees at the beginning of the fast. No change in temperature was noted until the twentieth day, when it increased nearly a degree, it reached ninety-seven degrees ten days later and remained at this standard thereafter. She also says that in a few subjects the temperature was so low that it could not be determined on a clinical thermometer, but "invariably normal individual average was reached before the end of the treatment."

Experiments upon starving animals show that the temperature remains normal through the fasting period and then begins to fall rapidly for from 2 to 6 days before death supervenes.

It is the rule, in chronic troubles, for the temperature to remain normal. Dr. Eales' temperature remained normal throughout his fast. Dr. Tanner's temperature dropped at the end of his fast, although he survived. This drop in temperature, both in man and in animals, undoubtedly marks the exhaustion of the body's reserve resources and the beginning of actual starvation.

I have had but one such case in my own experience, the sudden drop occurring on the 36th day of the fast. I broke the fast immediately and kept the patient warm with heat applied externally. He made a quick recovery and suffered no ill effects.

Carrington thinks that the fact that temperature falls to normal when above it and rises to normal when below it and that it reaches the normal point, in either case, just as the fast is completed and ready to be broken, is further proof that "fasting is a natural process, counseled by nature, with landmarks clearly defined, and but waiting to be recognized by man." This, it seems to me, is the only logical conclusion that can be drawn from the facts.

Despite the fact that the faster maintains normal temperature on a fast, or even has a slight rise in temperature, there is commonly a feeling of chilliness in a moderate temperature in which he ordinarily feels comfortable. This feeling of chilliness may be experienced, even when the bodily temperature is above normal, that is, when there is slight fever. We attribute this feeling of chilliness in individuals of normal or above normal temperature to decreased cutaneous circulation. Let a man strip nude in a cold room and remain there until he feels warm. Then let him walk nude into a warm room. Immediately, shivering results and he will feel cold.

It is well-known that heavy eaters are always complaining of the heat. They may be said to be constantly "feverish." Carrington suggests that the feeling of chilliness may be, in part, due to the absence of this feverishness. He suggests, also, that what is now regarded as normal temperature is a degree too high. The faster, the person on a fruit diet, the moderate eater, comfortable in summer, is likely to feel cold to the touch of the heavy eater.

Carrington records the case of a man whose temperature, by thermometric reading, was regularly, while eating, 2° F. below normal, yet he never felt chilly; but who on the twenty-third day of his fast, his temperature having risen to 97.8° F. (only .6° below normal), felt cold. He gives it as his opinion that the feeling of chilliness in this instance was due, in part at least, to decreased peripheral circulation—an anemia of the skin. But he also thinks that sharpened senses which, as we have seen, are rendered more acute in every instance of fasting, possess a keener perception to changes in body temperature.

We experience a sense of chilliness only when blood has been withdrawn from the skin; when, in other words, there is anemia of the skin, and we may actually be so chilly as to shiver on the hottest summer day. We may feel chilly while the thermometer shows our bodily temperature to be normal or slightly above normal. Geo. S. Keith, M.D., LL.D., records a case of a patient in which, he says: "The great peculiarity in the case was a chilliness coming on when he took anything like a meal." —*Fads of An Old Physician*, p. 168. This is somewhat a reversal of the chilliness seen in fasting, but it shows that the sensation of chilliness is not due to fasting, per se.

As pointed out before, whatever the explanation of the feeling of chilliness, it has nothing to do with the actual temperature of the body, which may actually be above normal. Susanna W. Dodds says of it: "In this cold paroxysm there is a rise in temperature (which the fever thermometer will detect) sometime before the chilling stage begins." —*The Liver and Kidneys*, p. 44.

In many cases, particularly of overfed individuals, we have what is called "famine fever" when a fast is entered upon. It is a slight elevation of temperature which may last from one to several days. I agree with Carrington that "it is, as in the case of all other diseases, a curative crisis, and should be regarded as a favorable sign, in consequence." Dr. Rabagliatti also regarded it as curative and added: "If we cannot fast without fever, it is because we have been previously improperly fed."

CHAPTER 17

Fasting and sleep

It is the usual thing for the fasting person to sleep no more than three to four hours out of each twenty-four hours, and this frequently causes worry. Three general causes for this sleeplessness are recognized: (1) It may be due to general nervous tension. The faster cannot sufficiently relax. (2) Sleeplessness is often due to a deficient circulation. The feet become cold and the faster finds it difficult to maintain warmth. A hot water bottle or jug placed at the feet will usually remedy this. (3) The fasting person does not require the usual amount of sleep. In a general sense, the amount of sleep one requires is proportioned to the quality and quantity of one's food. If you are comfortable and relaxed, you may be quite certain that you will sleep as much as you require.

In his narrative, from which I have previously quoted, Mark Twain records the case of one man who went without sleep for twenty-one days at a stretch, noticing during this period of fasting, no desire for sleep and no ill effects from not sleeping. Horace Fletcher frequently pointed out that when he ate less food he required less sleep. The sleeplessness and sluggishness that follow a heavy meal are well-known to everyone. If we are to be mentally alert, we must eat lightly or not at all. Such facts would seem to indicate that the digestion of large quantities of food is an exhausting process.

The faster that does not sleep is likely to fret and fuss about how long the nights are, but he does not feel the loss of sleep. It is true, of course, that all fasters who complain of not sleeping, like all other patients who declare that they never closed their eyes all night, sleep much more than they think they do. I have visited the rooms of fasters who complained of not sleeping and found them fast asleep, only to have they tell me the following day that they "never slept a wink all night."

A few patients sleep more while fasting than when eating. Insomnia victims are especially likely to do this. Fasting is perhaps the quickest and most satisfactory means of remedying insomnia, although there are cases in which it requires six to ten days to secure the sleep. Sinclair says, of his first fast: "I slept well throughout the fast."

I cared for one young man who slept sixteen hours out of twenty-four almost every day of thirty days fast. Another man, an asthmatic, slept almost day and night for days during and following the fast. But asthma cases, like insomnia cases, having lost much sleep, usually sleep much as soon as fasting brings relief from the dyspnea so that they can sleep.

Working during the fast:

On general principles working during a long fast is to be severely condemned. It has been done. It can often be done. But it should not be done. Perhaps the first fast of any length in which the faster worked was the twenty-eight days fast undergone by Mr. Milton Rathburn, a wealthy grain dealer, in 1899. Mr. Rathburn, who was a very fat man, took this fast to reduce upon the advice of Dr. Dewey and continued his daily work throughout the entire length thereof. According to the New York Press, of June 6, 1899, "he worked and worked hard. He came down earlier to his office and went away later than usual. He made no effort to save himself. On the contrary, he seemed determined to make his task as hard as possible."

Others have done this same thing and some of them were even more remarkable. In 1925, a weaver in Jersey City, N. J., fasted forty days and worked as a weaver throughout the time. On January 18, 1926, George Hassler Johnston, of New York City, a friend and co-worker of the author, began a fast which lasted thirty days, during which time he was unusually active. Mr. Johnston underwent this fast, under my supervision, purely as a publicity stunt and not because he was in need of a fast. He was an athlete of no mean ability and was in excellent physical condition at the beginning and at the end of the fast.

During the entire period of the fast, Mr. Johnston arose each morning at 5 o'clock and went to a radio broadcasting station, where he broadcasted three classes in exercises, each class lasting fifteen minutes. From here he usually walked a distance of twenty-five blocks to the offices of the McFadden Publications, where he entered upon his editorial duties. At 11:30 A.M. each day he visited one or the other of the three Physical Culture Restaurants in New York, where he remained until 2 P.M., meeting the people and answering their questions and giving advice upon fasting, diet and exercise. From the restaurant he would return to the office where, at 3 P.M., he conducted two classes, composed of McFadden employees, in calisthenics. After this he resumed his editorial duties, remaining at his desk until 5 P.M. During most of the fast he would walk home in the evening, a distance of 72 blocks, and spent his evenings at Madison Square Garden, watching the boxing and wrestling bouts. It was not until the end of the first week of the fast that he gave up his training at a down-town gymnasium and his track work—running.

This fast ended on the evening of Tuesday, Feb. 16, just 30 days after it had begun. On June 2, just three and one-half months thereafter, Mr. Johnston started from Chicago, in an effort to walk from there to New York without food. This stunt, I warned him against, but he made a brave effort and ended it June 20th at Bedford, Pa., having covered a distance of 577.8 miles in the 20 days.

This walk carried him over hills and valleys, through wind, rain, and the summer's heat and through crowds that flocked along the way. Handshaking, interviews, posing for pictures and making short health talks consumed almost as much of his energy as the walking. These often delayed him so that his walking on several days began late in the forenoon, although it often extended far into the night. I warned Mr. Johnston before he left to conserve his energies and predicted that he would go 20 days and no longer. He would have covered more miles in the same time he walked had he done more walking and less of other things, but he would still have ended on the 20th day.

This thing can be done, but it is damaging, even dangerous, and should never be undertaken. Gandhi, the Hindu Nationalist leader, who has probably fasted more than any other man in modern times, learned the necessity of conserving his energies while fasting. A painful mistake, which almost left him an invalid for life, taught him this lesson. It was while in South Africa that he took his second long fast, lasting fourteen days, that he foolishly imagined he could do as much work as while eating. On the second day after breaking the fast he began strenuous walking. This caused excruciating pains in the lower limbs, but he did the same the next day and for several days thereafter. The pains increased. His health was gravely injured by this and he was years in fully recovering from it. Of this he said: "From this very costly experiment I learned that perfect physical rest during the fast and for a time proportionate to the length of the fast, after the breaking of it, is a necessity, and if this simple rule can be observed no evil effects of fasting need be feared. Indeed, it is my conviction that the body gains by a well-regulated fast, for during fasting the body gets rid of many of its impurities."

This warning against working throughout a long fast does not apply to a short fast. I have on several occasions worked both at hard physical labor and at prolonged and exacting mental work for three or four days without food, and I have had hundreds of patients to do the same up to as high as nine days. But I do not think this should be prolonged beyond the tenth day, and where it is possible to absent oneself from work, it is best that all the time be spent in rest.

The practice pursued by many, of spending the whole day in activity, retards recovery from "disease." Conservation of energy should be the guiding principle.

Dr. Eales worked throughout his fast devoting eleven to twelve hours a day to the labors of his profession. He was very energetic during the whole time. Regular and frequent strength tests were made. The tests on the eleventh, sixteenth, twenty-first, twenty-third, twenty-fifth, twenty-ninth and thirty-first days of his fast showed his strength to be as great as at the beginning of the fast. The doctor reports that he could have competed in athletic work on thirtieth   day

CHAPTER 18

The effect of fasting on growth and regeneration

Growth is determined by two groups of causes—namely; the internal factor, of Growth Impulse, and the external factor, of Growth Control. The nature of the growth force or impulse, which is the real cause of growth, is wholly unknown. It is deeply rooted in the constitution of the organism and we say it is a predetermined, hereditary impulse to grow to a certain maximum under the most favorable conditions. This growth impulse is latent in the germ plasm and may be considered identical with life. The factors that control growth are pretty well known. These are food, water, air, warmth, sun light, or the absence of these. Internally we find, in the ductless glands, a remarkable chemical mechanism for regulating growth.

As before stated the growth capacity, which varies greatly with various species, is determined by heredity. Experiment seems to show that this impulse cannot be increased or completely repressed, although it is subject to considerable limitation. The interruption of nutrition by food deficiency or insufficiency or by inanition interferes with growth, but neither of these wholly suspends it. Judged by the gross weight of the body, growth may seem to be at a standstill, or even seem to be sliding backward. But this is very deceptive. A fasting organism that is losing weight and is consuming its reserves quite rapidly may still be growing.

Prof. Morgulis says the body "is a mosaic of interrelated parts, each, however, having its own growth history. The growth curve of one portion of the organism may be ascending while that of another has already reached the peak of its growth or indeed is on the downward course. Furthermore, the growth impulse of one may be great and that of another feeble. At times of plenty when there is enough nutriment to furnish building material for every part of the organism, the gross increase in weight is a good measure of the resultant growth; but it obscures the essential fact of the composite nature of the growth phenomenon. Walter's experiments with growing calves and Aaron's work on dogs illustrate this idea. These investigators discovered independently of each other that through chronic under-feeding they could keep their animals at a constant body weight but could not bring about complete standstill of the growing process. The part of the organism which at that phase of the development possesses the strongest growth impulse is potent to attract to itself whatever building material is available, and this not sufficing, will even encroach upon the reserves of other tissues. We witness, therefore, cataplasia or reduction of certain parts of an organism along with a progressive building up, or euplasia, of others. Such a condition has already been shown to exist in the salmon during the spawning season when these animals take no food sometimes for several months, and while all organs are used up, especially the muscles, in furnishing energy to the starving salmon, their gonads grow and develop luxuriantly. The young calves and dogs whose diet was thoroughly adequate in quality but not enough in amount, continued to grow though retaining a constant weight, but the growth was limited only to the skeleton. This increased both in size and mass, and as a result the animal actually grew in stature. Even the muscles were depleted of their stored material to satisfy the growth impulse of the skeleton."

The process of "robbing Peter to pay Paul" seen in these phenomena shows to a remarkable extent the power possessed by the body to distribute its supplies according to need, and thus preserve the integrity of the whole. If the robbing of Peter is not carried too far, no harm comes from it, for the consumed stores are readily and quickly replenished as soon as food is added. Growth seems to be independent of food in the sense that food is not the cause but only the material of growth. Dr. Morgulis finds in the phenomenon of regeneration a most remarkable exemplification of the fact "that the growth impulse of a particular organ may be sufficiently puissant to draw to itself nutriment and to infringe upon the reserves of the less active tissues and cause them to undergo cataplasia."

Properly conducted, fasting actually promotes growth. Thompson and Mendel found that a period of suppressed growth, due to under-feeding is followed by increased growth when better food is given, and that the acceleration of growth following this suppression, is ordinarily accomplished on less food than is consumed during a period of equal growth at normal rate from the same initial weight. Morgulis says: "It has been repeatedly emphasized that just as soon as an animal, which through acute or any other form of inanition lost weight, is given proper nourishment, it commences to grow at a spectacular rate and in a comparatively brief period regains all it had lost or even increases beyond the original level. The rapid gain in weight is a manifestation of a vigorous process of growth. There is not merely an accumulation of reserve substance, but a true growth in the sense defined previously. There is prolific cell multiplication, great expansion of the cells and a reaccumulation of reserves in the form of intracellular and intercellular deposits of products of their metabolism. Nitrogen is retained with an avidity characteristic of the young growing organism. Frequently, in a short span of time an increase of the body mass is accomplished, which required years of normal growth to bring about. The inanition has produced a rejuvenation of the organism. In the study of histological phenomena accompanying inanition, it has already been learned that except in the advanced stages (in the starvation period) there is scarcely any evidence of tissue degeneration. On the contrary, the cells remain intact though they lose a large portion of their substance. In the keen competition which reigns in the organism subjected to inanition the weaker and less essential parts of the cellular organism are sacrificed first, just as we have seen this to happen to the less essential parts of the entire organism. The more vital parts remain and the vitality of the cells and their vigor is thereby improved. This seems to be the rationale of the invigorating and rejuvenating effects of inanition. Biologically speaking, though the organism acquires no new assets it becomes stronger by ridding itself of liabilities. In the foregoing it has been pointed out that the cell-nucleus ratio changes in such a manner as to increase the preponderance of the nucleus. Morphologically, therefore, the cells composing the entire organism assume a youthful condition. They resemble more the embryonic cell in this respect, and this may account for the expansive growth which they display under the proper nutritive regimen."

Again, he says: "Further experiments performed with the salamander, demonstrated that the growth impulse and not the quantity of food consumed play the leading role. These experiments substantiated the idea that growth which ensues after a preliminary inanition is not unlike embryonic growth in its intensity. It is well to bear in mind that the reduced size of the cell, or rather the altered cell-nucleus ratio is probably in some way responsible for the vigorous growth process, and that the rejuvenescence of the organism is dependent upon this condition. Many years ago, Kagan observed that following 17 days of complete inanition rabbits gained 56 percent in weight on a diet which could just barely maintain a state of equilibrium in the normal condition."

Regeneration is common to a greater or lesser degree to all plants and animals. If man loses a fingernail, he quickly grows another, but even more remarkable examples of regeneration are seen in many animals, some of them being able to grow a new head, a complete new limb or an eye. In some worms a mere fragment of the body is capable of becoming a complete new worm. Many examples of this have been presented in a prior volume.

Prof. Morgulis says: "It is a remarkable fact that the starvating organism does not lose its regenerative power. An organism already much emaciated through prolonged inanition will draw upon its scanty reserves in the effort to renew a severed part of its body. The little flat worms, planaria, commonly found in stagnant waters, possess an extraordinary regenerative capacity. Morgan has shown that even in advanced stages of inanition, when the planarian has been reduced to a small fraction of its original size, the regenerative impulse is still sufficiently strong to reduce still further the much depleted tissues in rebuilding parts of the body which have been cut off. Of course, during inanition the missing organ does not regenerate as rapidly or as fully as in a well-fed animal. The important thing, however, is that inanition does not deprive the organism of its inherent regenerative impulse."

Discussing the fact that fasting does not interfere with the regeneration and growth of a new tail in the salamander, whose tail has been cut off, Morgulis tells us that, although the tail grows slower while the animal is fasting than the tails of animals not fasting, "when, after several weeks of starvation (fasting), the salamanders having in the meantime lost one-fourth their original weight, they were fed once more, the regeneration of the tail was immediately improved and in the course of time attained or even exceeded in length the tails which were cut off."

The Rhine salmon take no food from the time they enter the fresh water until their spawning season is over; a period varying from eight to fifteen months. The King Salmon of the Pacific coast, the largest and finest of the salmons, present an even more remarkable case of growth while fasting. They make a long and extremely exhausting journey upstream without food. There is evidence to show that they cease to feed before they begin their migrations upstream.

Salmon waste quite rapidly during their migrations, due not only to their vigorous activities, but to the rapid growth of their gonads. It has been estimated by Paton that 5 percent of the fat and 14 percent of the proteins of the wasting muscles of male salmon go to build up their rapidly growing testicles; while 12 percent of the fat and 23 percent of the protein of the muscles of the female go to build up the rapidly growing ovaries. The rest of the fat and protein that disappear from the muscles are used up in maintenance and work. Despite the rapid wasting of muscles in fasting salmon, Miescher maintains that not a fiber undergoes actual disintegration.

Our interest in the phenomena at this place is to point out the remarkable manner in which the body regulates its internal economy and distributes its stored supplies to various parts of the body as need arises. This ability to analyze and redistribute and re-synthesize the supplies on hand is our supreme guarantee that none of the vital tissues shall ever be damaged for lack of food, so long as the body's reserves hold out.

The continuance of growth while fasting and the rapid acceleration of growth after the fast, indicate very strongly that the body holds onto and uses to greater advantages those substances or qualities in food which are called vitamins and which are claimed to play such important roles in growth and regeneration of tissue. It may even be true that the body does not lose any of its stored supply of vitamins during the most prolonged fast. The complete lack of evidence to show that it does lose vitamins is as suggestive as is the positive evidence that fasting does not only not stop growth, but actually, accelerates it.

To investigate the impact of fasting on GH-mediated changes in substrate metabolism, insulin sensitivity, and signaling pathways.

DESIGN:

We conducted a randomized crossover study.

SUBJECTS:

Ten healthy men (age 24.3 +/- 0.6 yr., body mass index 23.1 +/- 0.4 kg/m (2)) participated.

INTERVENTION:

A GH bolus administered 1) postabsorptively and 2) in the fasting state (37.5 h). Skeletal muscle and adipose tissue biopsies were taken, and a hyperinsulinemic-euglycemic clamp was performed on both occasions.

MAIN OUTCOME MEASURES:

Metabolic clearance rate (MCR) of GH, substrate metabolism, and insulin sensitivity were measured. Biopsies were subjected to Western blotting for expression of signaling proteins and to RT-PCR for expression of suppressor of cytokine signaling protein 3 and IGF-I mRNA.

RESULTS:

Fasting was associated with reduced MCR of GH ($P < 0.01$), enhanced lipolytic responsiveness to GH, decreased insulin sensitivity ($P < 0.01$), and reduced IGF-I bioactivity ($P = 0.04$). After the GH bolus, phosphorylation of signal transducers and activators of transcription protein 5b (pSTAT5b) were observed in both conditions; however, the phospho-STAT5b/STAT5b ratio was significantly decreased in the fasting state (muscle $P = 0.02$ and fat $P = 0.02$).

CONCLUSION:

The combination of fasting and GH exposure translates into enhanced lipolysis, reduced IGF-I activity and insulin sensitivity, and blunted activation of the Janus kinase (JAK)/STAT pathway. Whether this change in signaling activity is related to the change in MCR of GH and/or the concomitant shift in the metabolic effects of GH merits future attention.

Fasting for more than 6 hours begins the cleansing phase. The cleansing phase is catabolic in nature in that it tears down old damaged cells. This process turns on brain autophagy, or "self-eating," in where the cells recycle waste material, regulate waste products and repair. These genetic repair mechanisms are turned on through the release of human growth hormone (HGH).

Intermittent fasting is one of the most powerful modalities for reducing inflammation; boosting immunity and enhancing tissue healing. This is one of the reasons why many people feel nauseated when they have infections. This innate mechanism is the body's way of influencing us to fast so it can produce the right environment to boost natural immunity.

HGH and insulin are opposites in function. HGH is focused on tissue repair, efficient fuel usage and anti-inflammatory immune activity. Insulin is designed for energy storage, cellular division and pro-inflammatory immune activity.

Insulin is the dominant player in this game. When conditions demand an insulin release (carbohydrate intake), HGH is inhibited. Additionally, too much protein or fat may not stimulate insulin but they will inhibit HGH release.

Studies have indicated that the disruption of neuronal autophagy results in accelerated neurodegenerative states throughout the brain. Elevated circulating levels of insulin reduce the amount of neuronal autophagy and cause metabolic problems as well as accelerated degenerative states.

Bouts *of intermittent fasting are essential for the brain to clean itself up* and drive new neurons and communication lines for optimal function.

The cleansing phase also acts like a slinky that is being spring-loaded for when the body moves into the building stage. It provides a sort of pre-load that allows the body to adapt in an incredible manner when it goes into the building phase. This enhances the neuronal connections and improves brain function.

Experts believe the intermittent fasting puts the brain cells under mild stress that is similar to the effects of exercise on muscle cells. The stress causes them to adapt and get more energy efficient. The body recovers from intense exercise through both the building and cleansing phases.

Brain-derived neurotrophic factor (BDNF) levels govern the formation of new neurons and the development of synapses and various lines of communication within the brain. Higher levels of BDNF lead to healthier neurons and better communication processes between these neurological cells. Low levels of BDNF are linked to dementia, Alzheimer's, memory loss and other brain processing problems.

Research has shown that bouts of fasting have a great anti-inflammatory effect on the entire body. Sufferers from asthma have shown great results as have preliminary reports on individuals with Alzheimer's and Parkinson's. Mattson and colleagues are preparing to study more details about the impact of fasting on the brain using MRI technology and other testing.

The best way to begin fasting is by giving your body 12 hours between dinner and breakfast every single day. This allows 4 hours to complete digestion and 8 hours for the liver to complete its detoxification cycle. After this is a standard part of lifestyle, try taking one day a week and extending the fast to 16-18 hours. Eventually, you may choose to do a full 24 hour fast each week.

During the fasting period it is great to drink cleansing beverages such as fermented drinks, herbal teas, water with infused super food extracts, water with lemon or apple cider vinegar, etc. These enhance the cleansing process by providing anti-oxidants and micronutrients that enhance healing while not interacting with insulin or HGH levels.

CHAPTER 19

Fasting in Drug Addiction

Addictions to drugs such as alcohol, cocaine, nicotine and caffeine are examples where fasting can dramatically reduce the often protracted withdrawal symptoms that prevent many people from becoming drug-free. Most people are surprised at how easy it is to quit smoking or drinking with the help of fasting.

Fasting was first used in alcoholism and later employed in other drug addictions; it may be well to begin with a brief study of this addiction. It is now everywhere recognized that the alcoholic is a sick man (or woman), but nowhere, it would seem, is the true nature of the illness recognized. Any form of drug addiction is an unintelligent seeking after "relief." Those who are comfortable seek no soothing poisons. Restless bodies and irritable nerves are soothed, often with the very occasion for the restlessness and irritability. The coffee user "relieves" her headache with more of the coffee that induced her headache in the first place. The morphine addict soothes his damaged nerves with more of the morphine that is responsible for their damage.

There is no drug-hunger, no craving for a poison of any kind, as is popularly supposed to exist in the victims of drug habits. The supposed craving for poison of any kind is a peculiar and unbearable nervousness arising out of exhaustion and injury. It is not a loud call for more stimulation (irritation) or more narcotization (depression)—nor yet a call for more poisoning, more injury, greater exhaustion—but a cry of distress. The real need is rest and a cessation of abuse. The "relief" that follows the repetition of the poison-dose is fictional and unreal.

Addicts take their beer and tobacco to soothe their distressed nerves. They feel weak and faint without them. They are just as weak and faint with them, but they are unconscious of the fact. The drug merely temporarily wipes out their awareness of their real condition. A man becomes irritable and cranky when denied his tobacco. The irritableness and crankiness are merely part of his general uneasiness—an uneasiness that has grown out of and is perpetuated by his habitual poisoning of himself.

That temporary respite from a sense of weakness and uneasiness, that temporary "relief" from misery and pain may be had from a re-narcotization of the nerves that are suffering from prior narcotization, leads the poor victim of the poison-vice to believe that his misery is a craving for his accustomed poison. This all adds up to the fact that the drug habit is the "relief" habit. Many drugs are said to be habit-forming. It is not the drug, but man that forms the habit. Man is, indeed, a habit-forming animal. For whatever reason he first takes the poison, he later takes it habitually as a means of escape from his intolerable suffering.

The development of the illness called alcoholism is so insidious that even the most thoughtful become enslaved to a remorseless habit, almost before they are aware of it.

Starting the use of alcohol, usually in youth, when the energy reserves of the body are so great that almost any amount of indulgence seems perfectly safe, the habit progresses to a chronic illness that seems hopeless to the helpless inebriate. Fettered by chains of his own forging, weakened in body, mind and will by the very indulgence that he would discontinue, suffering unutterably when he does not take his alcohol, he will often commit crime to get the "relief" he seeks.

The suffering of the alcoholic is so much greater than that which his drinking causes the members of his family that he does not hesitate to spend all his money for more alcohol and let the family suffer for want of food or other necessities. He finds temporary "relief" from his suffering by re-narcotizing himself with alcohol. He may have started drinking to drown sorrows that refused to stay drowned; he now drinks because he is miserable—a misery induced by his prior drinking—and he finds a fictional surcease from his unutterable misery in more of the narcotic that induced his misery. He is a sick man. He is profoundly enervated. His injured nerves will give him no peace.

When it is recognized that alcoholism is a chronic illness, it will be easy to understand how and why fasting may be of service in the condition. It is a period of rest during which the much abused organism undergoes much-needed adjustments and repairs and recuperates its wasted energies. When the fast is ended and the system has been freed of its accumulated toxins, and what is even more important, the nervous system has been restored to health; the supposed craving for alcohol is no more.

Alcoholism is an illness involving structural abnormalities. The thickening and toughening of the membranes of the mouth, throat and stomach are necessary defensive expediencies. Fatty degeneration of the liver or scleroses of the liver are, of course, late developments. When the alcoholic fasts the thickened membranes are removed and new membranes are formed. The new membrane of the mouth, tongue, throat and stomach will not be a thickened, seared one, impervious alike to foods and poisons, but a thin, delicate and sensitive one that permits full appreciation of the fine delicate flavors of foods.

Glands and nerves that have been lashed into impotency by overstimulation, rest into full functional power when given an opportunity. Renewal of their power can come in no other way. Will nerve energy be restored through rest? Just as certainly as a night of sleep will permit recuperation from the expenditures of the day. The abused organism will heal itself through rest as the broken bone will knit through rest. Do we deny rest to a broken bone, a wound, an ulcer? Do these need other means of healing? Can we deny that restorative cell-action resides within and that it operates best while the body is at rest?

Dewey said that the only remedy for alcoholism is "through a rest from all irritation from either alcoholics or food." He says of fasting in alcoholism: "the fast cure is one of the very easiest after the first three or four days, and even the most desperate old chronic can fast on for two, three, or even more weeks with only an increasing sense of comfort, and with no loss except disease and pounds. Was ever a cure for the alcoholic disease more rational, more in line with the very laws of nature?" He declared that there are only the fewest cases of chronic alcoholism so desperate, so long continued that a fast will not result in a new stomach, a repaired and renewed nervous system and a new outlook upon life.

Of this new outlook upon life, resulting from the emancipation of the man from his slavery to alcohol and of his renewed health, it may be well to take a brief glance. Dewey said to the alcoholic: "let me presume that for a whole month you have been absent from your homes are undergoing the rest (fasting) cure, aided by my encouragement, your homes the while having the 'peace be still' comfort you have not permitted for years. You will return to those homes saner men, and because of your clearer vision and soul power in reserve you will see far more in the countenance of that long suffering wife to love, honor and respect than you really were able to see in your days of food gluttony even before the alcoholic disease.

"And those children, as soon as they find that it is safe to be in the same house with you, will respond to your soul, born again, as the rose unfold under the favoring conditions of June. It will take them a little time to overcome fear of your attacks of emotional insanity, but in time they will get accustomed to the dazzling light where they have only found darkness and violence. As certainly will this be the result as you comply with the conditions."

Secret "cures" for alcoholism involve the expenditure of hundreds of dollars, weeks of absence from home and work, the introduction into the body of poisons (dangerous drugs) which are often worse than alcohol, and, usually, if not always, failure. The folly of trying to "cure" one poison addiction by resort to another poison should be apparent to all who read these lines. Occasionally the medical profession announces the discovery of a drug that will cure alcoholism or other drug addiction. As often as these poison-cures for poison-addiction are announced, they fail. Still the merry search for such a magic drug continues.

To the question: How long must I fast for alcoholism, Dewey replies: "Until you get into such comfort of body and mind that fasting will be a luxury. You will fast until there is a perfectly clean tongue and you feel capable of fasting unlimited. You will fast until there is a slight hint that some food of the nourishing kind is craved. Some of you will not get this felicity in less than a month, others sooner, and others will require even more time. The time is of no special account when cure is so certain and for such diseases as yours."

When the alcoholic has fully recovered from his illness and hunger has returned, no form of alcoholic drink will tempt him and should he attempt to drink some form, he will discover that he no longer "likes" it. It will bite and sting as it did when he first took it as a youth. He will be a free man again— no longer a slave to King Alcohol.

Let us look at tobacco next. Nicotinism, like alcoholism, is a chronic illness that is more or less willfully, although largely ignorantly cultivated. Young people usually begin the use of tobacco because it is "being done." It is the "proper thing." They must be in style, they must conform to the approved usages of the society in which they live and of which they are a part. Being in Rome, they must "do as the Romans do." Poor purblind fools! They know not what chains they are forging for themselves.

All that has been previously said about the use of alcohol, opium, etc., as a means of securing "relief" from uneasiness and distress, applies with full force to the use of tobacco. To chew or snuff, to smoke a pipe, cigar or cigarette, is to "relieve" distress—the distress of profound enervation. It is to re-narcotize the outraged nerves of the user of tobacco, to again cover up or hide from consciousness the true condition of the slave of Lady Nicotine.

Many tobacco-slaves try repeatedly to discontinue the use of the poison, but fail to succeed. They return to the poison-vice rather than endure the irritableness, grouchiness, "nervousness," and uneasiness that the prior use of tobacco has induced. They lack the determination to "tough it out," until the nerves have repaired themselves; they lack the will power to carry through; they are unwilling to bear the suffering, but return again and again to the fictional "relief" offered by another dose of their accustomed poison.

To such as these fasting is a God-send. It makes discontinuing the tobacco-vice easy, almost pleasant. Indeed, in but a few days the very taste of the weed becomes obnoxious. It is no uncommon complaint of the old smoker, after a thorough overhauling, that he cannot get a cigar of the right brand, or that he cannot find a cigarette that he likes. The difficulty is not, however, as he thinks, in the tobacco, but in his improved nervous system, and in the regenerated membranes of his mouth and nose. I have seen heavy smokers, who smoked half a life-time, after a fast, become so "sensitive" to the obnoxious fumes of tobacco that the odor of a cigar wafted to their nostrils from a block away was objectionable to them.

It should not be necessary to devote space to coffee, tea, chocolate and cocoa addiction. These poisonous substances (caffeine-containing drugs) are used by many millions of people for the same reasons that tobacco and alcohol are employed—to "relieve" distress. Caffeine is classed as a stimulant and is commonly employed by the enervated and weak to "sustain" them in their work or to keep them awake at night. Stimulation is wasteful of the energy of life, producing enervation. The headache, nervousness, unease, and suffering of the caffeine addict drives him, or her, to more of the same poison that produced his, or her enervation in the first place.

Other drug habits, such as the opium and morphine habit, the cocaine habit, the chloral habit, etc., are developed in much the same manner and follow much the same course in their development as the tobacco and alcohol habits. First resorted to in our search for "relief" from strain and tension, or from pain, or sleeplessness, or because of our mad search for thrills, the use of these drugs becomes a habit. This damages and enervates the nervous system to such an extent that the user is uneasy, uncomfortable, in pain and distress. He returns to his narcotic as a means of escaping from his intolerable suffering. Drug addiction is a phase of man's incurable escapism.

The drug addict uses no more intelligence in his search for "relief" from his exhaustion, unease and actual pain than does the sufferer with the jumping ache of a diseased tooth. His groaning nerves will not permit him to sleep and his distress cries out for "relief." "Relief" he will have if he has to die to get it. His resort to alcohol, or morphine, or cocaine, or other "relieving" poison is no more a matter of morals than the forceps of the dentist.

The opium and morphine habits are often the result of the use of these drugs by the physician in the treatment of some disease that can be more readily, and certainly more rationally cared for by Hygienic measures. The medical profession stands convicted of the crime of producing thousands of drug-addicts. As it pleads guilty to the charge, there seems to be no reason to labor the point. Cocaine using often becomes habitual as a result of using proprietary catarrh "remedies." Chloral and barbiturate addiction is a common result of the use of these drugs for purposes of inducing "sleep" in insomnia. Had the medical profession not taught mankind for ages that poisons are beneficent; these forms of poison addiction would be unknown.

McFadden's Encyclopedia of Physical Culture says: "Fasting is the most valuable of all forms of treatment for overcoming the pathologic condition of the body brought about by the habitual use of poison. Fasting gives the body an opportunity to readjust itself in a normal way and also hastens the elimination of any poison remaining in the system. The drug-fiend has lost his appetite anyway, and by means of a fast will regain a normal condition of the alimentary canal in a fraction of the time that would otherwise be consumed in the process. Especially the mind will clear and gain strength, and he will much sooner find himself in possession of the moral impulse and the will to fight his habit."

The digestive system and the nervous system of the dope addict are somewhat the same as those of the alcohol addict and from the same cause—habitual lashing with poisons. Rests—physical, mental and physiological—are the great needs. In a remarkably short time, the fasting patient finds his supposed "craving" for morphine or other poisons, has disappeared.

It is, of course, necessary to discontinue the use of the drug. Experience has shown just what we should expect on a priori grounds to be true, namely, that the abrupt withdrawal of all drugs at the very outset is far more satisfactory in the long run than any effort to gradually withdraw it. The "tapering off" process continues the injury and keeps alive the suffering that causes resort to the drug.

Violent reactions often follow the withdrawal of the drug. For this reason, it is essential to take great care of the patient. Mania following the withdrawal of morphine or opium, or delirium tremens following the withdrawal of alcohol is similar developments. They indicate the gravity of the injury to the nervous system and reveal how important and urgent is the need to get away from the use of the poison. It is much better, in cases of mania, to completely immerse the body of the patient in warm water for two to three hours, even if he has to be strapped in the tub, until his nerves become quiet, than to resort to even a small dose of the drug. A cold cloth or a cold pack should be placed on the head while the patient is thus immersed in the hot bath.

Bear in mind that these violent reactions soon cease as the patient fasts. With the gradual recovery of energy, repair of his damaged nervous system and regeneration of his membranes, the "call" for the "soothing" morphine, chlorate, cocaine, etc., grows so faint that it is easy to discontinue its use. Of the cases of morphinism I have assisted in caring for in this manner, not one, so far as I have learned, has ever returned to its use.

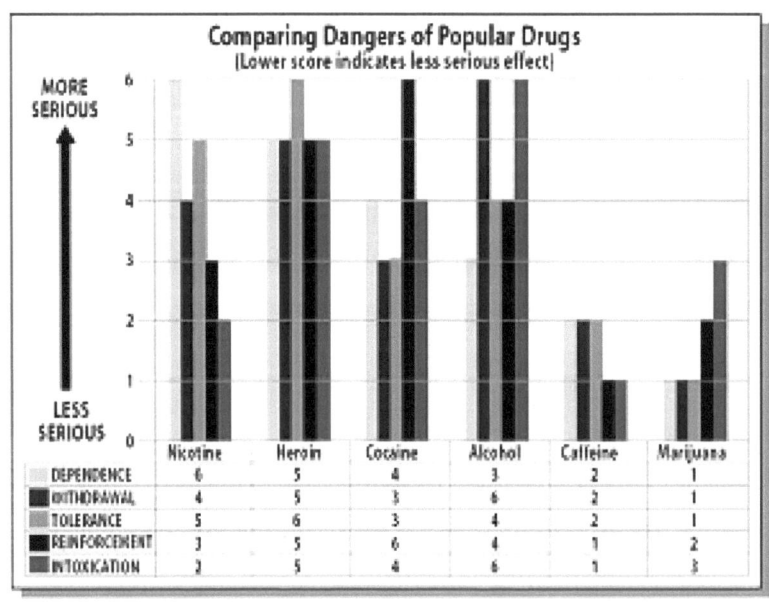

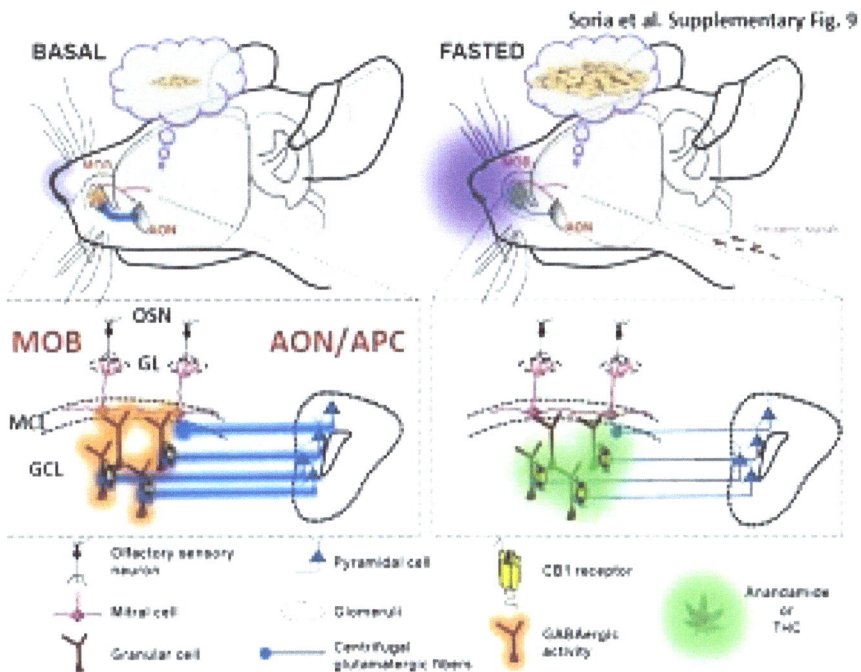

Diagram representing the mechanisms assumed to be involved in the (endo) cannabinoid effects on olfactory circuits in mice which have fasted.

AFTER-CARE OF THE ADDICT:

It seems necessary to point out that any return to the prior mode of living, after the fast, will reproduce a state of enervation and toxemia, thus giving rise to more suffering, which may tempt the "relief" seeker to again resort to the old "relief" measure. If he does this, he may again find himself in the grip of addiction. Only by first-class habits of living can any man guarantee himself against evils of all kinds. The eating habits of the former addict are of special importance.

The medical profession now says that drunkenness is a disease. They have not considered it so for any great length of time. On the other hand, the fact that it is a disease has long been recognized in Hygienic circles. I take the following statement from A History of the Vegetarian Movement by Charles W. Forward, published in London in 1878: "A remarkable instance of success in the treatment of intemperance by means of a vegetarian diet was that of Dr. James C. Jackson, of Dansville, N. Y. Writing in "The Laws of

Life," Dr. Jackson stated that "it is now twenty-five years since I took the position that drunkenness is a disease arising out of waste of the nerve tissue, oftentimes finding the center of its expression in the solar plexus or network of nerves that lies behind the stomach, and reflecting itself to the brain and spinal column by means of the great sympathetic. Since that time there have been under my care not less than a hundred habitual drunkards, some of them with such a desire for liquor that if they could get it they would keep drunk all the time; others having periodic turns of drunkenness, during the paroxysms of which they would remain drunk for a week or a fortnight at a time.

Every one of these persons was so far gone as to have lost all self-respect, character, and position, and many of them fine estates. In only two instances have I failed to give back good health and sobriety where these individuals have been under my personal management and direction; and of all the agencies that have been brought to bear upon them, save the psychological, none have proved themselves so effective as those of diet and bathing. It is morally and physically impossible for any man to remain a drunkard who can be induced to forego the use of tobacco, tea, coffee, spicy condiments, common salt, flesh meats, and medicinal drugs. If his diet consists of grains, fruits and vegetables, simply cooked, and he keeps his skin clean, he cannot, for any length of time, retain an appetite for strong drink. The desire dies out of him, and in its stead cooks up disgust. This disgust is as decidedly moral as it is physical. His better nature revolts at the thought of drinking, and the power in him to resist is strengthened thereby. The proof of this can be seen at any time in our institution, where we have always persons under treatment for inebriety. The testimony is ample, is uniform, is incontrovertible." And further on, Dr. Jackson declared, 'I have found it impossible to cure drunkards while I allowed them the use of flesh-meats. I regard animal flesh as lying right across the way of restoration. Aside from its nutrition, it contains some element or substance which so excites the nervous system as in the long run to exhaust it, to wear out its tissues, and to render it incapable of normal action'."

Note that he taught that both flesh and alcohol and other "stimulants" produce enervation—"waste of nervous tissue". Enervation is the basic fact in all addiction and to avoid re-cultivation of a drug addiction, it is essential that the individual so live that he does not enervate himself. While Dr. Jackson, in the foregoing, emphasizes addiction to alcohol, what he says is applicable to any drug addiction. It should also be stated that flesh eating is far from being the only, or the greatest enervating factor in the lives of our people. All sources of enervation should be studiously avoided. A well-nourished body, the energies of which are conserved by first-class habits, will not feel the "need" for stimulants and will not "need" to be "relieved" of discomforts and pains.

CHAPTER 20

The effect of fasting on blood

The blood diminishes in volume in proportion to the decrease in the size of the body so that the relative blood-volume remains practically unchanged during a fast. The quality of the blood is not impaired; indeed, an actual rejuvenation of the blood may occur.

Dr. Rabagliati pointed out that the first effect of the fast is to increase the number of red blood corpuscles, but if persisted in sufficiently long, decrease them. The increase of erythrocytes, during the early part of the fast, he regarded as due to improved nutrition resulting from a cessation of overeating. This increase in red blood cells has been repeatedly noted in anemia. The decrease is seen only after the starvation period is reached.

Prof. Benedict says: "Senator and Mueller in reporting the results of their examinations of the blood of Celti and Briethaupt noted an increase in the red blood corpuscles with both subjects. In a later examination of Succi's blood, by Tauszk, the conclusions reached were (1) that after a short period of diminution in the number of red blood corpuscles there is a slight increase: (2) that the number of white blood corpuscles decreases as the fast progresses; (3) the number of mononuclear corpuscles decreases: (4) the number of eosinophil's and polynuclear cells increases; and finally (5) that the alkalinescence of the blood diminishes."

Later experiments agree almost entirely with these results. The Carnegie Institute Bulletin, 203, pages 156-157 says: "The results of the above studies (of fasting) are conspicuous rather from the absence than the presence of striking alterations in the blood picture," and adds, "The final conclusions as to the effects of uncomplicated starvation on the blood to be drawn from the results of examination of Levanzin, are: In an otherwise normal individual, whose mental and physical activities are restricted, the blood as a whole is able to withstand the effects of complete abstinence from food for a period of at least 31 days (the length of Levanzin's fast), without displaying any essentially pathological change." Structural and morphological changes do not occur in normal blood cells during a fast.

Pashutin records the case of a man who died after four months and twelve days (132 days) without food and says that two days before death the blood contained 4,849,400 red and 7,852 white corpuscles in one cu. mm. Prof. Stengel says: "The blood in starvation preserves its corpuscular richness surprisingly, even after prolonged abstinence."

Fasting for only one week will increase the number of red cells in an anemic person. Medical and laboratory experimenters have conducted all their experiments on healthy men and animals; hence they have not been permitted to observe the regenerating effects of fasting upon the blood. Their statement that "human blood is relatively resistant during fasting" is true, but it does not tell the whole truth. Their statement that "there is a tendency to increase in the red cell count" is also true, but even this does not tell the whole truth.

Jackson says: "During human inanition, the erythrocyte (red cell) count is often within normal limits, but sometimes increased (especially in total inanition and earlier stages), or decreased (especially in chronic and late stages). In animals, the red cell count appears more frequently increased in the earlier stages of total inanition, often decreasing later. In hibernation, the erythrocyte count is variable." —Inanition and Malnutrition, -p. 239.

Normal blood contains from 4,500,000 to 5,000,000 and as high as 6,000,000 in healthy young men, red cells per cu. mm. and 3,000 to 10,500, with a probable average of 5,000 to 7,000 white cells per cu. mm.

Dr. Eales' blood was examined June 20, 1907, the first day of his fast, by Dr. P. G. Hurford, House Physician to Washington University Hospital, St. Louis. It showed the following:

Leucocytes 5,300 per cubic millimeter.

Erythrocytes 4,900,000 per cubic millimeter.

Hemoglobin 90%.

A blood test was again made on July 3, the 14th day of his fast, by Dr. S. B. Strong, House Physician, and Cook Gouty Hospital, which showed:

Leucocytes 7,000 per cu. mm.

Erythrocytes 5,528,000 per cu. mm.

Hemoglobin 90%.

It will be noted that the blood has materially improved on the fast.

A third examination of Dr. Eale's blood made by Dr. R. A. Jettis, of Centralia, Ill., on August 2, showed:

Leucocytes 7,328 per cu. mm.

Erythrocytes 5,870,000 per cu. mm.

Hemoglobin 90%.

A further improvement in the condition of his blood is here seen.

Laboratory investigators have reported an increase in the red cells of healthy fasters with a decrease in white cells. In anemia, fasting often results in an increase in the number of red blood corpuscles to more than twice their former number, with a concomitant decrease in the number of white blood cells. In a talk in Chicago a few years ago, Dr. Tilden said: "Cases of pernicious anemia taken off their food will double their blood count in one week." Dr. Weger reports a case of anemia in which a 12 days' fast resulted in an increase of the number of red cells from 1,500,000, to 3,000,000; hemoglobin increased fifty percent, and white cells were reduced from 37,000 to 14,000.

Wm. H. Hay, M.D., in his Health via Diet tells of caring for 101 cases of progressive pernicious anemia, during twenty-one years by fasting, correct diet and colonic irrigation. Of these 101 cases he says that 8 failed of initial recovery. Parts of the recoveries were made permanent by right living. Some of those who relapsed resorted once more to the fast and again recovered.

The first 13 cases of progressive pernicious anemia which Dr. Hay placed upon a fast recovered in from two weeks to longer. The fourteenth case, being in a dying condition when she arrived, did not recover. Dr. Hay says: "The blood during a fast undergoes no visible changes as to cell count unless markedly abnormal when the fast is begun in which case there is a return to normal." "For most of two weeks (in progressive pernicious anemia) the red, erythrocyte, count continues to fall before there is a regeneration in the blood-making organs; then gradually the microscopic picture begins to show round erythrocytes with regular edges, no crenations or irregularities, and soon there is noticeable increase in number of these with gradual disappearance of the adventitious cells present in the beginning.

"Not unusually there is a gain during the succeeding two weeks that brings the total back to the normal five million erythrocyte count, even though this may have been at, or below, one million in the beginning.

Von Norden says: "The blood atrophies." This is true of the *starvation* period, not *of fasting* proper. Much confusion will be avoided if the student will keep clearly in mind the fact that destructive changes occur only after the exhaustion of the body's reserves. Von Norden, Kellogg and others never tired of detailing the destructive changes that occur in the body during "starvation." Indeed, they were right in their details if they had used the term starvation properly. But they believed that the changes seen in starvation belong, also, to the fasting period. They made no distinction between the two processes. Later, investigators have corrected this old mistake, although few writers on the subject in our encyclopedias and standard works seem to have heard of this fact.

The decreased alkalinity due to prolonged fasting is often urged against it. It is contended that fasting produces acidosis. Fasting does not produce acidosis and the decreased alkalinity is never great enough, even in the most protracted fasts, to result in any deficiency "disease," unless the frequent cases of impotency are to be regarded as due to a loss of vitamins or mineral salts. The blood rapidly regains its normal alkalinity after feeding is resumed and no damage is done.

Mr. McFadden says: "It has been said that an acid condition of the blood, fluids and tissues (acidosis) is sometimes brought about by fasting. I cannot concede that this is ever the case, in true fasting. As a matter of fact, all the evidence seems to prove that as Dr. Haig expressed it, 'fasting acts like a dose of alkali.' If there is acidity in the system, fasting will remove it and restore the chemical balance of the system. Therapeutic fasting never created acidity, but on the contrary, removes that state when existing. Of course protracted starvation may do so, but then, whoever advised starvation.

"The medical as well as the general idea is that starvation begins practically immediately when meals are discontinued. The impression is that at once the blood and solid structures of the body begin to break down, that organic destruction has begun. Such is far from the case, as results have proved in scores (thousands) of cases. The vital cells of the organs and glands—those doing the active physical and chemical work of these parts—do not begin to disintegrate until actual starvation begins."

During a fast the body lives on its reserves. Starvation does not begin until these reserves are exhausted. What is more, these reserves contain sufficient alkaline reserves to prevent the development of so-called acidosis.

Dr. Weger says: "Varying degrees of acidosis were often in evidence during fasting. These we consider physiological. Except in very rare instances, the active symptoms are of short duration and easily overcome without interfering with or curtailing the fast." He describes the "symptoms of acidosis during a fast" as "lassitude, headache, leg and back ache, irritability, restlessness, redness of the buccal (mouth) mucous membrane and tongue, sometimes drowsiness, and also a fruity odor to the breath."

These symptoms develop at the beginning of the fast and grow less and less as the fast continues, until they cease altogether. If fasting produces acidosis the evidence should increase as the fast progresses. I believe that all of these symptoms may be explained without regarding them as evidences of acidosis. They result, I believe, from the withdrawal of the accustomed stimulation—coffee, tea, chocolate, cocoa, alcohol, tobacco, meat, pepper, spices, salt, etc., etc.—and are identical with these same symptoms when they develop in the man or woman who gives up coffee or tobacco, but who does not cease to eat. I do not think the "fruity odor" of the breath can be explained in this manner. However, in thousands of fasts I have conducted, I have never met with such a phenomenon—the breath in all cases being very foul and much like that of the fever patient or like the bad breath most people have, only much intensified.

Dr. Weger, himself, says: "*Fasting is not and cannot be the cause of acidosis*, for the symptom-complex of acidosis is quite common in full-fed plethoric individuals, in whom the makings of acidosis exist as a result of an over-crowded nutrition. It is true that symptoms of acidosis frequently occur and make patients decidedly uncomfortable during the early stages of the fast. However, these symptoms are due to excessively rapid consumption of the body fat—a catalytic action—and the checking of elimination because of sub-oxidation. In less than ten percent of such cases do these discomforts last more than three or four days? This indicates to us that the acidosis, as such, was a latent condition that would be excited into activity by any other equally potent provocative. This condition is analogous to a crisis which might occur in the form of an acute disease. The sicker one is made by a fast, the greater the need for it."

In general I agree with these words of Dr. Weger, but I have noted these supposed symptoms of acidosis in cases where there was no rapid breaking down of tissue, and in cases in which physical activity was sufficient to keep up normal oxidation and in which elimination was normal or super-normal. I do regard these symptoms as being part of a crisis and as beneficial in outcome. I have noted repeatedly that the more severe are these symptoms, the more benefit the patient receives from the fast and the sooner do these benefits manifest.

Fasting is important to all patients with pernicious anemia. Dr. Tilden remarked that "cases of pernicious anemia taken off their food will double their blood count in a week." Dr. Weger reported a less rapid increase and referred to one case in which hemoglobin increased 50 percent and white cells were reduced 50 percent on a 12 day fast. Dr. Hay's experience also was satisfactory, and he reported that of 102 pernicious anemia patients he treated with fasts of "generally two weeks or more" in duration, only eight failed of initial recovery. Some, who relapsed, due to an eventual return to poor dietary habits after the first fast, once again fasted and recovered. Dr. Hay stated that for most of the first two weeks of fasting, the blood count would continue to fall in some patients. But then the microscopic picture would begin to show "new round erythrocytes with regular edges, no crenations or irregularities, and soon there is noticeable increase in number of these with gradual disappearance of the adventitious cells present in the beginning." And during the succeeding days of fasting, the blood count would gradually return fully to normal.

CHAPTER 21

The effect of fasting on the immune system

Fasting allows the body to focus energy on cleansing and healing itself. According to these practitioners, fasting helps the immune system work more efficiently, allows more oxygen and white blood cells to flow through the body, helps the body burn more fat, helps increase energy, and allows other healing functions to improve. Some supporters claim that fasting by a person who has cancer can "starve" a tumor, leading to cell death.

Other illnesses and conditions proponents claim can be treated by fasting include acne, allergies, arthritis, asthma, non-cancerous tumors, digestive disorders, fever, glaucoma, headaches, heart disease, high blood pressure, inflammatory diseases, pain, polyps, and ulcers. Fasting is also promoted to rejuvenate the body, lose weight or help maintain normal body weight, increase longevity and sex drive, and to improve mental clarity, self-awareness, and self-esteem. It is also said to be helpful in quitting or cutting back on tobacco use, alcohol, caffeine, or non-prescription drugs. Some practitioners claim it can heighten spiritual awareness.

What does it involve?

Short fasts, lasting from 1 to 5 days, are often done at home. Other than drinking only water or juice, fasting can also require a lot of rest. Sometimes other methods of detoxification, such as liver flushes or enemas, are recommended as part of the regimen (*see also Juicing, Liver Flush, Colon Therapy*). Longer fasts require professional supervision and often take place at a spa, resort, or similar facility. Medical fasts are sometimes done at clinics or hospitals.

What is the history behind it?

Ancient cultures believed fasting could purify the soul. The belief that fasting can also purify or cleanse the body is a fairly modern idea, gaining popularity in the second half of the 20th century.

What is the evidence?

Available scientific evidence does not support fasting as a cancer treatment in humans. Some studies in animals have suggested that long-term calorie restriction—that is, consuming less than one's normal amount of calories each day—may slow the growth of certain tumors, but this is not the same as fasting. In fact, some animal studies have found that actual fasting in which no food is eaten for several days could actually promote the growth of some tumors. But more recent animal studies have showed some tumor growth slowed down during fasting.

A study published in 2012 looked at rodents with cancer who were given chemotherapy after 48 to 60 hours of fasting (they were given only water). They had better effects from the chemotherapy than rodents who ate normally before treatment, and in fact some who didn't get chemo had even improved. By itself, this does not mean the effect would be the same in humans. But studies are already under way to find out if fasting does help improve cancer treatment outcomes in humans.

In another report, 10 patients voluntarily fasted before (and some after) getting chemotherapy, and reported that their fatigue, weakness, and intestinal side effects were not as bothersome as when they got chemo while eating normally. Of note, they had different types of cancer and chemotherapy, and they fasted for different amounts of time, so it's hard to say whether these results will hold up with further testing.

In 2011, one research group looked at the available studies of calorie restriction and health in animals and humans, including the practices of religious fasting and other types of fasting. Their summary discussed animal studies in which restricting calories over the life span resulted in longer life and less chronic disease, including cancer.

They also reviewed animal studies that compared calorie restriction to alternate-day fasting, which means no food or very little food one day, alternating with eating as much as they wanted the next day, over long periods of time. (Alternate-day fasting can result in lower calorie intake, but often did not, as both humans and animals tended to eat enough on their "feast days" to make up for the fast days.) Some positive effects were found in long-term animal studies, but human studies of alternate day fasting have been much shorter and show fewer benefits.

A brief fast (usually 8 to 12 hours) is often advised by medical professionals in preparation for certain diagnostic tests. In this case, the fast helps to produce more accurate test results. Fasting may also be advised for a period of time before and after surgery, especially if digestive system organs are involved. This is mainly to ensure the stomach and bowels are empty during surgery. This is important to avoid getting stomach contents into the lungs, since anesthesia disables the usual protections, such as swallowing and coughing that keep a person from inhaling foreign matter into the lungs when he or she is awake. It also allows the intestines time to recover from anesthesia before reintroducing food.

As for reaching and maintaining proper weight, most experts recommend a combination of limiting portion sizes, choosing healthful foods, and being physically active instead of fasting.

Are there any possible problems or complications?

Fasting can have short-term side effects such as headaches, dizziness, feeling lightheaded, fatigue, abnormal heart rhythms, low blood pressure, and a fruity taste in the mouth. People who fast may have problems driving or operating dangerous machinery due to these effects. Fasting can also raise the risk of an attack in people with gout, and worsen symptoms of gallstones. Longer-term fasting can interfere with the immune system and vital bodily functions and can damage the liver, kidneys, and other organs. Fasting can be especially dangerous in people who are already malnourished, such as those with some forms of advanced cancer. Death results when fasts outlast the body's supply of stored fuel or energy.

Dry fasting (no fluid intake) can quickly result in dehydration and death over a period of days, with the length of time varying by person and situation. Factors such as extreme heat, exertion, or illness can shorten it to a few hours.

Women who are pregnant or breast-feeding should not fast. People taking certain medicines can have problems with absorption, as well as changes in drug action and side effects.

Relying on this type of treatment alone and avoiding or delaying conventional medical care for cancer may have serious health consequences.

Fasting cycles:

Prolonged fasting forces the body to use stores of glucose, fat and ketones, but it also breaks down a significant portion of white blood cells. Longo likens the effect to lightening a plane of excess cargo.

During each cycle of fasting, this depletion of white blood cells induces changes that trigger stem cell-based regeneration of new immune system cells. In particular, prolonged fasting reduced the enzyme PKA, an effect previously discovered by the Longo team to extend longevity in simple organisms and which has been linked in other research to the regulation of stem cell self-renewal and pluripotency—that is, the potential for one cell to develop into many different cell types. Prolonged fasting also lowered levels of IGF-1, a growth-factor hormone that Longo and others have linked to aging, tumor progression and cancer risk.

"PKA is the key gene that needs to shut down in order for these stem cells to switch into regenerative mode. It gives the OK for stem cells to go ahead and begin proliferating and rebuild the entire system," explained Longo, noting the potential of clinical applications that mimic the effects of prolonged fasting to rejuvenate the immune system. "And the good news is that the body got rid of the parts of the system that might be damaged or old, the inefficient parts, during the fasting. Now, if you start with a system heavily damaged by chemotherapy or aging, fasting cycles can generate, literally, a new immune system."

Prolonged fasting also protected against toxicity in a pilot clinical trial in which a small group of patients fasted for a 72-hour period prior to chemotherapy, extending Longo's influential past research.

"While chemotherapy saves lives, it causes significant collateral damage to the immune system. The results of this study suggest that fasting may mitigate some of the harmful effects of chemotherapy," said co-author Tanya Dorff, assistant professor of clinical medicine at the USC Norris Comprehensive Cancer Center and Hospital. "More clinical studies are needed, and any such dietary intervention should be undertaken only under the guidance of a physician."

"We are investigating the possibility that these effects are applicable to many different systems and organs, not just the immune system," said Longo, whose lab is in the process of conducting further research on controlled dietary interventions and stem cell regeneration in both animal and clinical studies.

The study was supported by the National Institute of Aging of the National Institutes of Health (grant numbers AG20642, AG025135, P01AG34906). The clinical trial was supported by the V Foundation and the National Cancer Institute of the National Institutes of Health (P30CA014089).

In the first evidence of a natural intervention triggering stem cell-based regeneration of an organ or system, a study in the June 5 issue of the Cell Stem Cell shows that cycles of prolonged fasting not only protect against immune system damage—a major side effect of chemotherapy—but also induce immune system regeneration, shifting stem cells from a dormant state to a state of self-renewal.

The study has major implications for healthier aging, in which immune system decline contributes to increased susceptibility to disease as people age. By outlining how prolonged fasting cycles—periods of no food for two to four days at a time over the course of six months—kill older and damaged immune cells and generate new ones, the research also has implications for chemotherapy tolerance and for those with a wide range of immune system deficiencies, including autoimmunity disorders.

"We could not predict that prolonged fasting would have such a remarkable effect in promoting stem cell-based regeneration of the hematopoietic system," said corresponding author Valter Longo, Edna M. Jones Professor of Gerontology and the Biological Sciences at the USC Davis School of Gerontology and director of the USC Longevity Institute.

Prolonged fasting forces the body to use stores of glucose, fat and ketones, but it also breaks down a significant portion of white blood cells. Longo likens the effect to lightening a plane of excess cargo.

During each cycle of fasting, this depletion of white blood cells induces changes that trigger stem cell-based regeneration of new immune system cells. In particular, prolonged fasting reduced the enzyme PKA, an effect previously discovered by the Longo team to extend longevity in simple organisms and which has been linked in other research to the regulation of stem cell self-renewal and pluripotency—that is, the potential for one cell to develop into many different cell types. Prolonged fasting also lowered levels of IGF-1, a growth-factor hormone that Longo and others have linked to aging, tumor progression and cancer risk.

"PKA is the key gene that needs to shut down in order for these stem cells to switch into regenerative mode. It gives the OK for stem cells to go ahead and begin proliferating and rebuild the entire system," explained Longo, noting the potential of clinical applications that mimic the effects of prolonged fasting to rejuvenate the immune system. "And the good news is that the body got rid of the parts of the system that might be damaged or old, the inefficient parts, during the fasting. Now, if you start with a system heavily damaged by chemotherapy or aging, fasting cycles can generate, literally, a new immune system."

"While chemotherapy saves lives, it causes significant collateral damage to the immune system. The results of this study suggest that fasting may mitigate some of the harmful effects of chemotherapy," said co-author Tanya Dorff, assistant professor of clinical medicine at the USC Norris Comprehensive Cancer Center and Hospital.

A new study in the *journal* Cell Stem *Cell* shows that cycles of prolonged fasting prompts the human immune system to rejuvenate hematopoietic stem cells from dormancy to a state of self-renewal. Hematopoietic stem cells, which reside in bone marrow, are those from which all other blood cells are derived. The findings represent the first academic confirmation of a natural action prompting stem regeneration of an organ or system.

One of the authors of the study, Valter Longo, a professor at the University of Southern California (USC) Davis School of Gerontology, labeled the effect "remarkable." When the human body is starved, he said, it tries to conserve energy. One of the ways it does this is to "recycle" immune cells, including those which may be damaged.

Humans in the six-month clinical trials fasted regularly for between two and four days over a six-month period. It has been known that fasting forces the body to use glucose, fat and ketones it has held in storage. Now, with the new study, it is also known that three-day fasts break down a meaningful portion of white blood cells. Longo compares the effect to ridding an airplane of extra baggage.

Not eating for long periods lowered white blood cell counts significantly. Simultaneously, it is as if "a regenerative switch" was flipped for hematopoietic stem cells, thus providing the first, important step in the generation of blood and the regeneration of immune systems. Professor Longo says that once this "OK" is issued, stem cells proliferate, and rebuilding of the entire, critically-important immune system commences.

The new discovery will likely be helpful to cancer patients who are doing chemotherapy treatments and their inevitably damaged immune systems. It could also be helpful for elderly people, whose immune systems are less effective and for whom the fighting off of common diseases is more difficult.

Longo's team noticed that, in both humans and animals, white blood cell counts decreased when associated with fasting. Each cycle of fasting depletes white blood cells in the body, thus triggering changes that begin the stem cell-based regeneration of new immune system cells. Toxicity was also seen as being protected against with fasting.

Tanya Dorff, a co-author of the study and an assistant professor at the USC Norris Comprehensive Cancer Center and Hospital, noted that chemotherapy causes significant incidental damage to the human immune system, and the study suggests that fasting may allay some of the damage caused by the chemotherapy. More studies are needed, she cautioned, and suggested that any such attempts to fast should only happen with a physician's supervision. Cycles of fasting can literally generate a new immune system, she said.

Whereas most abnormal growths that have disappeared while fasting have been benign tumors, a considerable number have also been diagnosed as malignant.

Dr. Shelton states that he has seen cancer patients "become free from all pain in twenty-four hours to three days when the drugging was discontinued and all feeding stopped.

"He also reported actual recovery of one case which had previously been diagnosed as cancer in as little as three days of fasting. Of course longer fasts are required in most instances of suspected cancer, and Dr. Hazzard recorded a case in which 45 days of fasting were required before recovery was complete.

Another experienced worker in this field, Dr. Rasmus Alsaker, supervised "the return to health of many individuals diagnosed as having cancer of the stomach" with the fasting treatment, although he did not discount the possibility of mistakes of diagnosis in these cases.

As a rule the chances of recovery from cancer depend largely upon the stage of the disease and the history of previous therapeutic treatment. In early cancer, which has not been treated with surgery nor radiation, and which has not involved the prolonged use of pain-killing drugs, the prognosis is frequently favorable.

The slow absorption of the neoplasm of cancer can then be expected in many cases.

In certain cases there is not complete absorption, though further growth may be checked.

If the neoplasm of cancer has been broken with exploratory or therapeutic surgery, with release of cancer cells to other parts of the body, and if tissues have been weakened with extensive X-ray therapy, the chances of recovery are markedly lower.

If, in addition to these adverse factors, the patient has been kept

Under a state of sedation until he is suffering more from the effects of drug addiction than cancer, we find the least favorable prognosis. However, even when cancer is in its hopeless stage, fasting may be considered of some value in reducing pain and bringing the patient to a more comfortable end than could otherwise occur.

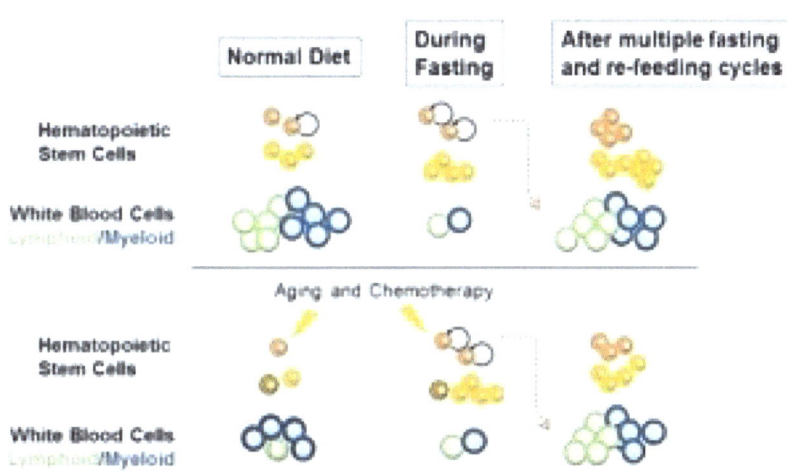

During fasting the number of hematopoietic stem cells increases but the number of the normally much more abundant white blood cells decreases. In young or healthy mice undergoing multiple fasting/re-feeding cycles, the population of stem cells increases in size although the number of white blood cells remain normal. In mice treated with chemotherapy or in old mice, the cycles of fasting reverse the immunosuppression and immunosenescence, respectively.

CHAPTER 22

Contraindications to Fasting

List a number of contra-indications for fasting. These need clarification. They follow:

(1) Fear of the fast on the part of the patient. Fear may kill where the fast would be of distinct benefit. If fear of the fast can be overcome there is no reason why it should not be instituted.

(2) Extreme emaciation. In such cases a long fast is impossible. A short fast of one to three days may often be found beneficial, or a series of such short fasts with longer periods of proper feeding intervening may be found advisable.

In extremely emaciated patients I do not favor pushing the fast to the return of hunger, but favor a process of careful nursing with one or more short fasts. Whereas, Carrington points out, that such patients may die before the return of hunger, I am convinced from experience, that with a careful nursing program and but limited fasting, these patients may be restored to health in many cases that would otherwise die.

I have repeatedly fasted such cases, even for as much as twenty-two days at a time; always with distinct benefit. Indeed, the fast is often the only thing that will enable these cases to overcome their emaciation.

(3) In cases of extreme weakness or of extreme degeneration. Even in many such cases a series of short fasts, as mentioned before, may often be beneficial. In the latter stages of consumption and cancer, the fast can be of no value except to relieve the patient's suffering. It may prolong life a few days. Fasting is of distinct benefit in the earlier stages of both of these conditions, however.

Great weakness is not always a danger signal; rather it may often prove to be a "false alarm." More often than otherwise, weakness signifies poisoning or a crisis. It is essential that the weakness be considered in union with all other symptoms present. Indeed, this is true of all the danger signals. No one of them, considered by itself, constitutes an evidence of real danger. Carrington regards periods of great weakness that are often seen in fasting patients as crises, or periods of great physiological change going on in the body. He says that "the fact that hitherto weak hearts are actually strengthened and cured by fasting proves conclusively that any such unusual symptoms, observed during this period, denote a beneficial reparative process, and not any harmful or dangerous decrease or acceleration, due to lack of perfect control by the cardiac nerve." In this connection I may add that I have never seen a death from "heart failure" during a fast, although I have seen many crippled hearts make complete recoveries during a fast. Prostration and weakness are part of the process we call disease, and are not due to the lack of two or three meals. Hence it is that, as the patient returns to normal, strength returns even when no food has been eaten or digested.

It has been pointed out in the preceding pages that great weakness is not necessarily a bar to fasting; that it is in such cases that we often see the greatest gains in strength.

(4) In cases of inactive kidneys accompanied by obesity. In such cases it is said that the tissues may be broken down faster than the kidneys are able to eliminate them. This I doubt. I know of no reason why the tissues of the body should be used up faster at this time than at other times. It is true that there is increased elimination during the fast but this is not so great as to constitute a great burden upon the kidneys. I have repeatedly fasted cases of Bright's "disease" and cases of kidney stone, kidney abscess and myelitis with distinct benefit in all such cases.

(5) In marked "deficiency diseases." Some advocates of fasting do not advise fasting in these conditions; but hold that, since they are due to food deficiencies, these patients need a changed diet rather than a fast.

It was shown in previous pages that fasting is distinctly beneficial in rickets, anemia and other deficiencies, and that a failing appetite in these conditions plainly indicates the need for a brief fast. It should also not be overlooked that in all deficiencies there are toxic states that must be overcome before the best of diets can do its perfect work. Deficiency is not always due to faulty diet. It may be due to impaired nutritive machinery and function, from a variety of causes. Physiological rest is frequently the first essential to recovery in such cases.

(6) Difficult breathing. This symptom is sometimes seen in two types of cases; namely, nervous cases and cases of heart impairment. In nervous cases it constitutes no warning of danger. In heart cases, it should cause a careful watching of heart action. Should this show signs of weakening; the fast should be terminated at once.

I have fasted many cases, with nothing but benefit, which would not have been placed on a fast by others who employ this measure. I have continued fasts in cases where others would have discontinued the process, with no development in any case of any of the troubles or evils against which we are so frequently warned.

I have fasted cases for more than twenty days who were advised by Dr. Hazzard not to fast more than five days. I have fasted cases that Dr. Hazzard had previously placed on lemon juice and honey rather than on a fast. Fear of legal consequences, should something go wrong, prevents many advocates of fasting from using it to its greatest advantage.

We have the development of medicine in general in the treatment of ulcers, and can ill ulcers fasting if he does not complain of any symptoms were assessed his health by gastroenterologist before Lent, but requires the use of drug ulcers, consult a physician task until the patient feels stable condition, because fasting is working to increase gastric acid and the effect of the acid in the absence of food is so severe and lead to the erosion of the mucous membrane, and thus avoids the complications which will be mentioned later.

- Prevents fasting for patients who develop ulcers acute or active «sharp pain + vomiting» - a modern occurrence - with the knowledge that pain in the upper abdomen not diagnosed as ulcer active it was found that 70% of those who suffer from pain in the abdomen do not have signs of ulcer active «must see a doctor»

- It also prevents fasting for patients with ulcers do not respond to treatment or who have bleeding ulcers in a short period of less than three months, for example, and also patients who have undergone surgery modern and them ulcer complications of infections and bleeding in the stomach or the duodenum or obstruction or perforation ulcers and also in elderly patients with ulcers.

Patient liver and gallbladder:

The liver is an important member of the human body, and its significance lies in that it is the largest member in terms of size and consists of several cells and greater number of complex processes in terms of bio-chemical, and rids the body of toxic substances and harmful.

Therefore, we find that liver disease depending on the place of infection; biliary channels hepatocytes, liver tissue and blood vessels also differ in their treatment, which ranges from a change in the pattern of food to medication to surgery.

A balanced diet is important in general for the treatment of liver diseases, particularly chronic or late.

Fasting patient with liver and gallbladder diseases as mentioned above must to consult his doctor before fasting in the assessment of his state of health, and often a liver patient can fasting if the disease is chronic in its early stages and it is complications or accompanied by other diseases prevented from fasting, such as diabetes and others.

Here are some situations that prevent fasting for liver patients:

1- Patients with chronic diseases and late stages and patients with complications such as cirrhosis and liver failure and hepatic coma and inflammation of the membrane proton in the abdomen and severe fatigue.

2- Should be considered therapeutic drugs, especially if they are taken at frequent intervals, and also patients who use diuretics, because these drugs make the patient lose a large amount of fluids and salts, should the patient be compensated directly, and this harms used in the treatment of hospitalization associated with some diseases of the liver, so they must be eaten.

3 - Patients with bleeding esophageal varicose were treated by endoscopic injection are susceptible to both sores in the esophagus or stomach, here are the best to be non-fasting.

With the exception of the above-mentioned cases can to fast safely, only in coordination with the doctor before fasting.

There are cases in which it is well to proceed cautiously and in which the inexperienced person should not attempt to conduct a fast; but in general there is seldom any such thing as a contra-indication to fasting, just as there is seldom or never a contra-indication to any other form of rest.

The liver after the fast:

Fasting is but a means to an end. It is a cleansing process and a physiological rest which prepares the body for future right living. It is, therefore, necessary that the work begun by the fast be continued and completed after the fast.

Most fasting advocates advise great care in breaking the fast and in subsequent feeding and then feed terribly. Dr. Eales, for example, followed his thirty days fast with an exceedingly bad diet. He broke his fast on Horlick's Malted Milk and was soon eating such meals as the following: "Glass of malted milk with raw egg, and ate one poached egg later." Dinner (6 P.M.) "Two soft-boiled eggs, glass of milk, little rice and strawberries." He also mentions that he "had a cup of coffee" with some friends.

Dewey's personal diet consisted chiefly of meat, fish, eggs, milk, pastries and bread, with but few vegetables, these chiefly of the starchier varieties. He was opposed to acid fruits, declaring they all contain potash which decomposes the gastric juice and that "there is never any desire for acid fruits through real hunger, especially those of the hyperacid kinds: they are simply taken to gratify the lower sense—relish." Acid fruits can be "taken with apparent impunity" "only by the young and old who can generate gastric juice copiously."

The demoralizing influence of all acids, fruit acids included, exerted upon gastric secretion, is undoubted. But this does not necessitate abstaining from acid fruits and does not prove them to be harmful. It only calls for eating them alone. Dr. Dewey knew nothing of food combining. He referred to apple eating as converting the human stomach into a cider mill and declared that "by their ravishing flavor and apparent ease of digestion, apples still play an important part in the 'fall of man' from that higher state, the Eden without its dyspepsia." It was his notion that if we "eat from hunger" and not "from mere relish," we would eat right without much attention being given to what we eat. While there is perhaps more truth in this than is generally recognized, it is, unfortunately, not absolutely true.

Pearson lived for the first week after his fast was broken on about 2 oz. of sweet chocolate, 2 oz. of peanuts and one and sometimes 2 chocolate malted milks, from the soda fountain, a day.

Tanner tells us of his own overeating, that after his fast (he was dyspeptic before going on the fast) he ate "sufficient food in the first twenty-four hours after breaking the fast to gain nine pounds, and thirty-six pounds in eight days, all that I had lost." If I can judge by the results of over-eating after a fast, that I have observed, Tanner's gain in weight was a puffy, water-logged mass of material that cannot by any stretch of the imagination be called healthy or desirable. His uncontrolled eating was a dangerous procedure and he was in luck to escape with his life. It would not be wise for others to attempt this foolish stuffing. The inability of the undisciplined individuals of our country and age to control themselves means that they should not undertake to feed themselves at all after a fast. They should be controlled by a man of experience.

It will be quite obvious to the student of diet that the style of eating followed by these men must inevitably undo much of the benefits derived from the fast.

In many quarters it is the almost invariable practice to follow a fast with a milk diet. It is my invariable practice not to follow the fast with such a diet. The milk diet undoes much of the benefit derived from the period of abstinence. Dr. Hazzard also condemns the milk diet following the fast. Sinclair noted that very frequently the milk diet disagrees with people, and says: "Inasmuch as there is nothing that poisons me quite so quickly as milk, I had to look farther for my solution."

He further says concerning his experience with milk, "I was never able to take the milk diet for any length of time but once, and that after my first twelve-day fast. After my second fast it seemed to go wrong with me, and I think the reason was that I did not begin it until a week after breaking the fast, having got along on orange juice and figs in the meantime. Also I tried on many occasions to take the milk diet after a short fast of three or four days, and always the milk has disagreed with me and poisoned me. I take this to mean that, in my own case, at any rate, so much milk can only be absorbed when the tissues are greatly reduced; and I have known others who have had the same experience."

It is quite true that after a long fast one is capable of absorbing large quantities of milk, but there still remains the question of why one should do so. Why go on the fast in the first place if it is to be followed by worse gluttony than ever?

Dewey was opposed to special exercises. Rabagliati was of the opinion that exercises are not necessary to health and life, and that the ordinary movements supplied by the ordinary business of life are physiologically sufficient for this purpose. This is obviously not true in many occupations. Besides, exercise serves many purposes and few, if any, of the occupations of modern life supply all of the body's needs for exercise.

If we are to continue to enjoy good health after a fast, proper diet, adequate and fitting exercise, sunshine, fresh air, mental poise, rest and sleep and freedom from devitalizing habits are essential. The length of time through which the results of a fast will last depends upon how one lives after the fast.

"Diseases," when treated by drug and serum methods, frequently recur after they appear to be cured. I am frequently asked if this is true of fasting-"cured" cases. To answer this question correctly, it is necessary that the reader distinguish between "regular" methods of treating "disease" and fasting. Drugs and serums succeed only in suppressing the symptoms of "disease," so that an apparent cure often results. But suppression of symptoms does not constitute a real cure. Fasting does remove the internal causes of "disease." It purifies the organism. A cure by this means is a true cure, and is not merely a forced suppression of symptoms.

But fasting cannot make one "disease"-proof. If a certain mode of eating and living makes a man sick once, it can do so a thousand times if he returns to it. When a man has been cured through fasting, if he resumes over-eating and wrong eating and sensuality and inebriety, excesses, dissipations and other forms of wrong living, he will again build "disease" in his body. It may be the same condition or some other, but he is certain to evolve some form of "disease" if he does not live rightly after his body has been cleansed. If, like the Biblical so that was washed, he returns to his wallowing in the mire, he cannot help but become dirty again and will require another bath. But if he will live as he should live, he may be fully assured that he will not have a recurrence of his troubles. Once "disease has been "cured," by natural methods, the person cannot again have the "disease "without building it all over again.

Sinclair likens a man who needs a fast "every now and then," to the man who spends his time sweeping rain water out of his house, instead of repairing the roof. If there is need for you to fast at frequent intervals, this is because you're eating and living habits are wrong. If you give up drinking you will not need to be sobered up at frequent intervals.

Enervation, established as a chronic state following enervating habits, lowers and perverts functioning of the organs of the body, some functions being weakened more than others. If we do not build enervation and toxemia by taxing the organism to the very limit, no pathology will develop. Lighten the toxic over-load with which the organism has been burdened, cultivate conservative habits of living, guide the mind into new channels of thought, poise and control the emotions, and getting well and remaining well is no longer a game of chance.

After the fast, the diet should be both unrefined and uncooked to as great an extent as possible.

In view of the present chemical and radioactive contamination of our physical environment, including our food supply, this step is not certain to provide the perfect nutrition that was once attainable, but it will give the best nutrition possible within the framework that exists. While not ideal, this is still sufficient for the purposes in question. For some patients after fasting, an adequate food stock may be available and an excellent nutritional basis may be established.

Others will doubtless deviate from the optimum nutritional standard, but all can keep the general goals of scientific nutrition in mind and endeavor to follow them as much as possible.

Though correct diet is important as a permanent phase of living after the fast, it is especially so for the first few weeks or months, when the body is regaining normal weight.

During this period a very high percentage of nutriment is being absorbed from the food, and if the new protoplasm being built is to be healthy and biologically adequate, the source material must be of high quality.

If reconstruction is made entirely from the same foods which rendered the body ill in the first place, the eventual advantages of the fast may be virtually nullified.

Once the body weight is stabilized, and maintenance is the only requirement, the food will cease to be so vital a determining factor, though it will still affect the health in a very definite manner and should be selected with care.

So long as correct nutrition is maintained after the fast do the proper foods remain enjoyable and satisfying? There is generally no desire or craving for highly refined foodstuffs, and even the want for alcoholic beverages and tobacco may have disappeared. If change is then made, however, back to a more conventional mode of nutrition, this ceases to hold true and many of the old desires return.

Appetite is chiefly a result of habit, and though it can be normalized by fasting, it can again be restored to a condition of abnormality and perversion, insofar as the associated intake of food supplies, in adequate measure, the nutritional needs of the body.

CHAPTER 23

Heightening your awareness

A wonderful thing about fasting is that it puts an interval between the behavior that you are accustomed to and the behavior that you aspire to. We tend to be creatures of habit, and the ways that we are accustomed to eating and living feel as natural to us as breathing. That is why it is so difficult for people to stop bad habits. But fasting brings your present lifestyle to an abrupt halt. It gives you an opportunity to pause, reflect and decide how you are going to conduct your life afterwards. This enables you to make a break with your past and set off in a new, more positive direction.

There is nothing routine about eating after a fast. Each meal is a celebration. After fasting, you tend to be very conscious about what you are eating, and why. Fasting heightens your awareness as well as your appreciation for food. By fasting, we learn to eat with reverence.

It is the non-doing aspect of fasting that enables us to make behavioral stopping and pausing and interrupting our usual patterns, as we learn to take more conscious control of ourselves.

There is no better way to stop a vicious cycle of self-destructive behavior than by fasting.

Fasting thus must be recognized only as a means of promoting the remedy of disease and the creation of health. It is not a method of maintaining health. This depends, as it always has, with both man and animals, upon the general hygienic factors of proper nutrition, sunlight, exercise, pure air, etc.

The purpose of fasting is basically therapeutic, and in this sense it not only meets the requirements of most patients, but is perhaps the most effective measure ever to be employed.

Clearly the extraordinary value of fasting has not been recognized by the professions of healing as a whole.

In spite of the careful scientific work done with fasting by physiologists, biologists and physicians, and the almost universal recommendation of the method by these people, Islam is built on five pillars. Each represents a unique utility, an institution, if you will, through which the believer builds his relationship with the Creator and the creation. Of all the pillars of Islam, none is more special than Fasting. While there may be an appearance of eye service, or show, in all other pillars—prayer, Zakat, Hajj, and even the word—there is no such possibility in fasting. The only One who knows that you are really abstaining is Allah. It is easy to pretend to be fasting; while in hiding, you may eat or drink. Thus, fasting is considered a special worship, as Hadith reports from the Messenger of Allah have detailed.

"O ye who believe! Fasting is prescribed to you as it was prescribed to those before you, that ye may (learn) self-restraint,-" (Surah Al Baqarah 2:183)

It has been reported by the way of Abu Hurairah that the Prophet reported that Allah said in a Hadith:

"'All the deeds of Adam's sons (people) are for them, except fasting which is for me, and I will give the reward for it.' Fasting is a shield or protection from the fire and from committing sins. If one of you is fasting, he should avoid sexual relation with his wife and quarreling, and if somebody should fight or quarrel with him, he should say, 'I am fasting.'

The Prophet added, 'By Him in Whose Hands my soul is' The unpleasant smell coming out from the mouth of a fasting person is better in the sight of Allah than the smell of musk. There are two pleasures for the fasting person, one at the time of breaking his fast, and the other at the time when he will meet his Lord; then he will be pleased because of his fasting." [Sahih Bukhari: Book # 31: Hadith #128]

Among the points this incisive hadith revealed is that fasting is Allah's. Certainly, there is only one reason why a believer will put himself or herself through this trying physical exercise that—to seek the pleasure of Allah. The fast is the single most important device to test the belief, faith, of the believer and the depth of his sincerity and commitment to the concept of the Oneness of Allah.

The hadith also states that fasting is a shield, an armor protecting the believer from sinful acts. Do you not know that nourishment is the first culprit in the propagation of sins? For when you eat, the blood flow increases considerably, and the energy level increases, making it easier for Satan (evil) to use your own energy level to tempt you to commit sins. In another hadith, the Prophet states:

"Satan (evil) runs in the circulatory system of the son of Adam in the same way blood circulate in our system; so tighten his passages with hunger." (Bukhari/Muslim)

Now you see why fasting becomes a shield. Fasting enables the believer to guard against his arch enemy. It also helps him against human evil by putting the patience and perseverance gained from fasting into use with forbearance and forgiveness of the attacker—that is, of course, when the safety of one's life is not involved. Otherwise, in this case, Quran allows the believer to repel evil without transgression.

References

1- Herbert M. Shelton, Fasting Can Save Your Life, Natural Hygiene

Press, Inc., Chicago, IL, 1964.

2-Arnold De Vries, Therapeutic Fasting, Chandler Book Co., Los Angeles, CA, 1963.

3- Herbert. M. Shelton, fasting Therapeutics, translation and publication, Rashid Dar, 1987, Damascus, Beirut.

4-William F. Ganog. Review of Medical physiology. 15th Edition 1991. Appleton & Lange, Los Altos, California.

5-The British journal Nature Saturday 11/25/2000 AD.

6- J. Hywel Thomas and Brian Gilliham, Will's, Biochemical Basis of Medicine, 2nd Edition (1989), London.

7-Goldhamer D.C., Alan, The benefits of fasting, true north health center, May 30, 2010.

8-jockers, Dr. David, Increase brain function with proper fasting techniques, Natural health 365, Fri. Feb. 1, 2013.

9-The journal of clinical endocrinology and metabolism, Impact of fasting on growth hormone signaling and action in muscle and fat 2009 Mar; 94(3):965-72. Doi: 10.1210/jc.2008-1385. Epub 2008 Dec 9, PMID:

19066303[PubMed - indexed for MEDLINE].

10-Parker-pope, Tara, Regular Fasting May Boost Heart Health, The New York Times, April 4, 2011.

11-saudi medical journal, Impact of fasting in Ramadan in patients with cardiac disease, 2005 Oct; 26(10):1579-83., PMID: [PubMed - indexed for MEDLINE].

12-Intermountain Medical Center, Routine periodic fasting is good for your health, and your heart, study suggests, May 20, 2011.

13-Al-Oballi Kridli Suha PhD, RN, Health Beliefs and Practices of Muslim Women During Ramadan, MCN, The American Journal of Maternal/Child Nursing, August 2011, Volume 36, Number 4 Pages 216 – 221.

14-Saudi journal of kidney diseases and transplantation, Ramadan fasting and transplantation: Current knowledge and what we still need to know, vol.21, issue 3,2010, page 417-420.

15-Wu, Suzanne, Fasting triggers stem cell regeneration of damaged, old immune system, university of southern California news, June 5, 2014.

16-American cancer society, fasting, Medical Review: 02/24/2012.

17- Baskin, Gregory. Fasting Generates a New Immune System, The Telegraph, USC news, university Herald, June 13, 2014.

18- Nizal Sarraf-Zadegan, MD; Mahmoud Atashi, MD; Gholam A. Naderi, PhD; Abdoul M. Baghai, MD; Sedighe Asgary, PhD; Mohammad R. Fatehifar, MS; Hossien Samarian, MS; Maryam Zarei, BS,(THE EFFECT OF FASTING IN RAMADAN ON THE VALUES AND INTERRELATIONS BETWEEN BIOCHEMICAL, COAGULATION AND HEMATOLOGICAL FACTORS)., Annals of Saudi Medicine, Vol 20, Nos 5-6, 2000.

19- An Interview with Dr. Joel Fuhrman: Master of Fasting, Copyright 2008, Track Your Plaque., Special report.

20- J P McCann and W Hansel, Relationships between insulin and glucose metabolism and pituitary-ovarian functions in fasted heifers, Biology of reproduction, the Society for the Study of Reproduction2014

21- Natural Instinct Healing, Fasting for fertility, 12 Dec, 2012.

22-Ames, john, Importance of intermittent fasting, Medica Health&Therapy center.

23-(The Elliott P. Joslin Research laboratory, the department of medicine and surgery, Harvard medical school, the cardiovascular unit, the peter bent Brigham hospital, and the Diabetes foundation, Inc., Boston, Massachusetts), Brain metabolism during fasting, The Journal of Clinical Investigation, Vol. 46, NC. 10, 1967.

24- Karmananda Saraswati, Dr. Swami, MB, BS (Syd), Psychophysiology of Fasting, Yoga magazine, May 1981.

25- R. G. Cridland, M.D., (Fasting Facts & Myths), International natural hygiene society (INHS), 2003.

26-Dickerson, Lauren, MD, (CHANGING RISK FOR INJURY: AMERICA'S PRESCRIPTION ADDICTION), Well true, MD, APRIL 29, 2014.

27-(Prescription Drug Abuse: A Fast-Growing Problem), NIH Medline Plus, fall 2011 Issue: Volume 6 Number 3 Page 21.

28-(Addictive Properties of Popular Drugs), DrugWarFact.org, © 1998-2014, Common Sense for Drug Policy.

29- Routine periodic fasting is good for your health, and your .., http://www.sciencedaily.com/releases/2011/04/110403090259.htm_br (accessed October 4, 2014).

30- Monitoring blood pressure -, http://www.marylandbirthcenter.com/patiented/articles/monitoring_blood_pressure_000294.htm_br (accessed October 4, 2014).

31- Soil and Health Library, http://www.mdsarequacks.com/books/devries.fasting.pdf_br (accessed October 4, 2014).

32- How Does Heart Disease Affect Women? - NHLBI, NIH,
http://www.nhlbi.nih.gov/health/health-topics/topics/hdw/_br (accessed
October 4, 2014).

33- Heart Scan Resource Center - Track Your Plaque,
http://www.trackyourplaque.com/library/fl_06-023fuhrman.asp_br
(accessed October 4, 2014).

34- WEAR IT to Win it! - Transformyx, Inc,
http://www.dynasite.net/s3web/1001932/Docs/innovation_handbook.pdf
?S=1001932&M=171&SM=&SC=999999&P=Y&U=&SS=&ModuleTyp
e=135&subfile=vars&pl=100&SP=/s3web/1001932_br (accessed
October 4, 2014).

35- THE EFFECT OF FASTING IN RAMADAN ON THE VALUES
AND ..,
http://www.2muslims.com/books/2discoverislam_com_002.pdf_br
(accessed October 4, 2014).

36- The effect of fasting in Ramadan on the values and ..,
http://www.researchgate.net/publication/6539148_The_effect_of_fasting
_in_Ramadan_on_the_values_and_interrelations_between_biochemical
_coagulation_and_hematological_factors_br (accessed October 4, 2014).

37- Effects of Fasting on the Brain, Nervous & Endocrine Systems,
http://www.thehealersjournal.com/2013/04/15/fasting-effects-healing-
the-brain-nervous-endocrine-system/_br (accessed October 4, 2014).

38- Detox and Cleansing for Preconception Care,
http://katereardon.com.au/detox-and-cleansing-for-preconception-
care/_br (accessed October 4, 2014.

39- Fasting for fertility | Natural Instinct Healing,
http://naturalinstincthealing.com/fasting-for-fertility/_br (accessed
October 4, 2014).

40- The Monthly Transmitter (July 2012) - Parkinson's disease ..,
http://www.parkinsons.va.gov/Consortium/cfiles/July_12_Transmitter.a
sp_br (accessed October 4, 2014).

41- Decapeptyl SR 22.5mg - X-PIL,
http://xpil.medicines.org.uk/ViewPil.aspx?DocID=24161_br (accessed
October 4, 2014).

42- Relationships between insulin and glucose metabolism and ..,
http://www.ncbi.nlm.nih.gov/pubmed/3518823_br (accessed October 4,
2014).

43- June 21, 2014 is World ALS Day! Come and join us in the event ..,
http://www.mndoxfordshire.org/wp/wp-
content/uploads/2014/06/GORONfor-ALS_Oxford.pdf_br (accessed
October 4, 2014).

44- Mineral, Protein and Vitamin Deficiency in Causing Hair Loss,
http://www.healthclop.com/mineral-protein-and-vitamin-deficiency-in-
causing-hair-loss/_br (accessed October 4, 2014).

Contents

INTRODUCTION

CHAPTER 1: Fasting in history

CHAPTER 2: Chemical and organic changes during fasting

CHAPTER 3: Fasting means therapeutic

CHAPTER 4: Fasting and modern scientific research

CHAPTER 5: The effect of fasting on gastroenterology

CHAPTER 6: Fasting and diabetic patients

CHAPTER 7: The effect of fasting on heart health

CHAPTER 8: The effect of fasting on the brain and the nervous system

CHAPTER 9: The effect of fasting on the endocrine glands

CHAPTER 10: The effect of fasting on eye diseases

CHAPTER 11: The effect of fasting on respiratory diseases

CHAPTER 12: Fasting and infectious diseases

CHAPTER 13: Fasting and patients with urinary tract problems

CHAPTER 14: Fasting and transplantation

CHAPTER 15: Fasting during pregnancy and lactation

CHAPTER 16: Fasting and body temperature

CHAPTER 17: Fasting and sleep

CHAPTER 18: The effect of fasting on growth and regeneration

CHAPTER 19: Fasting in drug addiction

CHAPTER 20: The effect of fasting on blood

CHAPTER 21: The effect of fasting on the immune system

CHAPTER 22: Contraindications to fasting

CHAPTER 23: Heightening your awareness

References